Praise for
re/entry: a guide for nurses dealing with substance abuse disorder

"Authors Crowley and Morgan know what recovery is about! Their book *Re/Entry: A Guide for Nurses Dealing With Substance Use Disorder* is an excellent resource for nurses in any stage of recovery and for colleagues and friends who care about nurses in recovery. This practical guide intimately walks the reader through what is important to know and reflect upon related to substance abuse support, treatment, recovery, and reentry. Written with compassion and insight and with vignettes sprinkled throughout, this text is an important, meaningful addition to the nursing literature."

–Linda L. Smith, ARNP, MN, MDiv, CARN-AP
Chief Executive Officer, Florida Intervention Project for Nurses

"This book is a must-read for any nursing professional and others who have been dependent on drugs or who have dealt with family, peers, coworkers, or others who have or have had substance use disorders. Health professionals generally have easier access to substances; thus addictions are common in this population. Substance use disorder crosses all walks of life, all professions, and, in nursing, all practice settings. This book takes one on a personal journey—leaving the medical model of addictions treatment and detoxification and moving toward introspection to gain and maintain recovery. I applaud the authors for creating and providing this journey."

–Al Rundio, PhD, DNP, RN, APRN, CARN-AP, NEA-BC
Associate Dean for Post-Licensure Nursing Programs & CNE
College of Nursing & Health Professions, Drexel University
President, International Nurses Society on Addictions

"*Re/Entry* is full of real-world, down-to-earth guidance for the recovering nurse or anyone who knows someone struggling with a substance use disorder. The authors expertly mix humor, hope, and many tried-and-true-techniques for the road to recovery to help illuminate this disease and diminish the fear so generally associated with it."

–John Southworth, CADC, NCAC, ICAADC, BRI-II
Program Coordinator, Idaho Program for Recovering Nurses

D1569437

"*Re/Entry* provides a clear, step-by-step guide to what happens when a person seeks assistance for a substance abuse disorder. The book is a source of insightful support to the person struggling with the disorder and will be an invaluable resource for family, friends, and employers as they journey to understand and support the recovery process."

–Ben Murray, MN, RN
Former Substance Abuse Nurse Investigator, Reentry Facilitator,
Nurse Manager, and Administrator

"I can't say enough about the work that Crowley and Morgan have done in their book: *Re/Entry: A Guide for Nurses Dealing With Substance Use Disorder.* As a recovering addict, former emergency room nurse, former CRNA, peer assistance advisor, and now chemical dependency counselor, I will use this book as a resource and recommend it to every nurse I know who is dealing with the disease of chemical dependence. Crowley and Morgan have provided hope for nurses dealing with SUD and a step-by-step guide on how to proceed with treatment, recovery, and reentry to the profession they love. Thank you for an outstanding guide and a much-needed resource for the profession!"

–Jack Stem, CDCA
CEO, Peer Advocacy for Impaired Nurses, LLC

"I would highly recommend this book to any nursing leader who manages health care workers. Having been a leader and nursing executive for more than 25 years, I have often dealt with issues of substance abuse and addiction. This book does a very effective job of illustrating the experience of individuals coping with substance abuse issues along with the challenges that they face in their recovery. Hearing real-life stories of recovery is essential in understanding their experience. This is a must-read for health professionals!"

–Ellen Talbott, MSN, RN, CPHQ, CENP
Vice President of Patient Care Services/CNO, McLaren

"*Re/Entry* is about recovering from addiction, from the nursing perspective. It provides all the basic information a nurse needs to face his or her substance abuse problem and begin living a clean and sober life. Crowley and Morgan share their vast experience and knowledge in a conversational way that makes *Re/Entry* a quick and easy read. Their advice about how to overcome resistance is sure to be welcomed by nursing managers as well."

–Annabeth Elliott, MSN, RN
Director of Investigations, Idaho Board of Nursing

Doody's
D.F. 100
2018
+ebook

re/entry

a guide for nurses dealing with substance use disorder

Karolyn Crowley, RN; Carrie Morgan, BA

WY
87
.C953
2013

Sigma Theta Tau International
Honor Society of Nursing®

Copyright © 2014 by Karolyn Crowley and Carrie Morgan

All rights reserved. This book is protected by copyright. No part of it may be reproduced, stored in a retrieval system, or transmitted in any form or by any means, electronic, mechanical, photocopying, recording, or otherwise, without written permission from the publisher. Any trademarks, service marks, design rights, or similar rights that are mentioned, used, or cited in this book are the property of their respective owners. Their use here does not imply that you may use them for similar or any other purpose.

The Honor Society of Nursing, Sigma Theta Tau International (STTI) is a nonprofit organization whose mission is to support the learning, knowledge, and professional development of nurses committed to making a difference in health worldwide. Founded in 1922, STTI is a global community of nurse leaders. Members include practicing nurses, instructors, researchers, policymakers, entrepreneurs, and others. STTI's 486 chapters are located throughout Australia, Botswana, Brazil, Canada, Colombia, Ghana, Hong Kong, Japan, Kenya, Malawi, Mexico, the Netherlands, Pakistan, Portugal, Singapore, South Africa, South Korea, Swaziland, Sweden, Taiwan, Tanzania, the United Kingdom, the United States, and Wales. More information about STTI can be found online at www.nursingsociety.org.

Sigma Theta Tau International

550 West North Street

Indianapolis, IN, USA 46202

To order additional books, buy in bulk, or order for corporate use, contact Nursing Knowledge International at 888.NKI.4YOU (888.654.4968/US and Canada) or +1.317.634.8171 (outside US and Canada).

To request a review copy for course adoption, e-mail solutions@nursingknowledge.org or call 888. NKI.4YOU (888.654.4968/US and Canada) or +1.317.634.8171 (outside US and Canada).

To request author information, or for speaker or other media requests, contact the Marketing Communications director of the Honor Society of Nursing, Sigma Theta Tau International at 888.634.7575 (US and Canada) or +1.317.634.8171 (outside US and Canada).

ISBN: 9781938835155
EPUB ISBN: 9781938835162
PDF ISBN: 9781938835179
MOBI ISBN: 9781938835186

Library of Congress Cataloging-in-Publication data

Crowley, Karolyn, 1955- author.
  Re-entry : a guide for nurses dealing with substance use disorder / Karolyn Crowley, Carrie Morgan.
    p. ; cm.
  Guide for nurses dealing with substance use disorder
  Includes bibliographical references.
  ISBN 978-1-938835-15-5 (alk. paper) -- ISBN 978-1-938835-16-2 (ePub) -- ISBN 978-1-938835-17-9 (PDF) -- ISBN 978-1-938835-18-6 (MOBI)
  I. Morgan, Carrie, 1957- author. II. Sigma Theta Tau International, issuing body. III. Title. IV. Title: Guide for nurses dealing with substance use disorder.
  [DNLM: 1. Nurses--psychology. 2. Nursing--standards. 3. Rehabilitation--psychology. 4. Return to Work--psychology. 5. Substance-Related Disorders--rehabilitation. WY 87]
  RT41
  610.73--dc23
                        2013023338

First Printing, 2013

Publisher: *Renee Wilmeth*
Acquisitions Editor: *Emily Hatch*
Editorial Coordinator: *Paula Jeffers*
Cover Designer: *Rebecca Batchelor*
Interior Design/Page Layout: *Rebecca Batchelor*

Principal Book Editor: *Carla Hall*
Development and Project Editor: *Kate Shoup*
Copy Editor: *Tonya Maddox Cupp*
Proofreader: *Andrew Kimmel*
Indexer: *Jane Palmer*

Dedication

We dedicate this book to you as you move through life's obstacles back to your beautiful true self.

Acknowledgments

Most importantly, we want to acknowledge those who cared for us before we could care for ourselves. Some of you are named Matt, Delray, John, and Jeanette.

We are vastly grateful to the peer support group participants and alumni who contributed recovery, wisdom, and hope. You know who you are. You are on every page of this book.

Our appreciation to the many who gave their time and expertise to this book and who continually contribute to making this a better world. Our particular gratitude to Jeanette Flood, First Step, CADC, OT; John Southworth, CADC, NCAC, ICAADC; Ben F. Murray, RN, MSN; Cynthia (Cindy) Clark, RN, PhD, ANEF, FAAN; Sandra Evans, Executive Director, Idaho Board of Nursing; Mark H. Broadhead, M.D., ABPN certified addiction psychiatrist; Ted Burgess, LCSW; Janet Edmonds, MSN, RN, Director for Professional Compliance IBN; Kathy Russell, JD, MN, RN; Nancy J. Brent, RN, MS, JD; managers, J. D. and D. R.; Kevin G., EAP; Dennis Wedman HR; Debbie Ketchum, MAOM, BSN, RNC, C-EFM; Ellen Talbott, MSN, RN, CPHQ, CENP Sue Magnusson, RNC; Sandy and Brad for research assistance; and all those who remain anonymous. In the future, we hope there will be more hospital managers who feel free to speak out. In the meantime, we send you support as you work behind the scenes.

Thank you for rapid responses and valuable contributions, Dr. Cynthia Clark and Dr. Don Morgan.

Thanks to Michael, for your love, support, and encouragement. We also thank our families, friends, and sponsors for providing volumes of love, growth opportunities, and support. Don and Pat, the writing retreat was a luxury! Robert, Arlene, and John, your offers were golden. For sheer spiritual and physical fortitude, cleaning up our messy drafts, and nourishing our bodies while keeping the midnight oil burning, thank you, Lois Morgan.

About the Authors

Karolyn Crowley, RN, is founder of Insight Support Groups, a recovery program for nursing professionals. Crowley has been sober and in recovery for more than 15 years. In 2001, after embracing sobriety and finishing the Idaho Board of Nursing's alternative-to-discipline program, she was asked to facilitate a nurse support group under the auspices of the board. In 2009, she founded Insight Support Groups, a recovery program that emphasizes the establishment of a healthy lifestyle as a key strategy for maintaining sobriety.

Crowley has been a registered nurse since 1985. Her nursing experience includes clinical practice as well as nursing education and health care research. The majority of her nursing experience has been in the ER and in labor and delivery. She has also worked in such diverse areas as flight nursing and infertility medicine. Currently, she is certified in the specialty areas of inpatient obstetrics and electronic fetal monitoring, as well as advanced cardiac life support (ACLS) and neonatal resuscitation.

Crowley lives in Boise, Idaho, with her husband, Michael, and a small menagerie of animals. She spends her time outdoors running, horseback riding, and skiing when she is not working. She also enjoys traveling and scuba diving whenever possible. To learn more about Crowley and Insight Support Groups, go to www.insightsupportgroups.com.

Carrie Morgan, BA, is a recovery coach, business consultant, speaker, and writer. Her expertise for recovery coaching comes from combining 14 years of coaching and consulting expertise with recovery principles. Morgan exploits her lifelong curiosity of personal transformation and 19-plus years of recovery to accompany her clients and support groups on the journey from addiction toward self-mastery. She also trains professional coaches in her Intentional Living Model (ILM). Her hybrid approach blends recovery principles, emotional intelligence (EQ), energetic integrity, and the dictum of constant and never-ending improvement as a path to access personal fulfillment and professional success. The foundation for her work is based in the concept of ego versus essence. In all her work, she helps her clients to identify and manage their egoic perceptions in order to access their essential brilliance.

One of Morgan's favorite activities is running the trails around Boise, Idaho, with her sidekicks, Shaggy Maggie and Neely. She also likes getting out of her comfort zone and learning more about gardening, softball, snowboarding, and tennis. Laughing with family and friends rates high on her list of things to do. She can't wait for her next trip. For more about Morgan's notions and vocation, visit www.carriejmorgan.com or join others on Facebook at https://www.facebook.com/carriejmorgansintentionalliving.

Table of Contents

Foreword

When it comes to substance abuse—that is, the abuse of alcohol and/or drugs—health care professionals, including nurses, are particularly vulnerable. This is no doubt in part because the industry brings together a perfect storm of opportunity, motive, and means. In the United States alone, some one in 10 nurses—an estimated 300,000 in all—suffer from substance use disorder (SUD). Of particular concern with nurses is prescription drug abuse.

It's very possible that you work with, care about, or even are a nurse suffering from SUD. If so, what should you do? As a critical first step, I suggest you read *Re/Entry: A Guide for Nurses Dealing With Substance Use Disorder*. This extraordinary book brings the critical knowledge about chemical dependency in the nursing profession together with the essential how-to-do-it tools for successful reentry. This much-needed source of illumination should be read by every nursing student, colleague, and educator. Most importantly, it should be read by members of every board of nursing. These individuals and organizations face important decisions about allowing recovering nurses back into clinical practice and monitoring the progress of these reentering nurses toward stable recovery.

It's true that there is no known cure for SUD, but recovery is possible. The goal of this book is to offer a light in the dark—to show support for nurses who have supported others. The text is remarkable in a number of ways. Perhaps most notably is the fact that it speaks the language of recovery—not just recovery from SUD, but emotional and spiritual recovery from the often devastating comorbidities as well as a shame-based definition of self. While the text certainly stands up to academic rigor, it also seeks to impart information in a conversational manner to help comfort those suffering from substance abuse disorder and to urge them to get the help they so desperately need.

The personal stories of many recovering nurses and their struggles to return to clinical resonate throughout the book. They are utilized as superb case studies that illustrate the steps from impairment to recovery. Many of these stories are quite moving, although the frustration of dealing with a faceless bureaucracy at times is very apparent. This is often a reflection of the insane variability a recovering RN may have to contend with, depending on his or her state of residence.

In summary, this is a priceless addition for all of us who struggle with providing effective support to our colleagues in recovery and for people who themselves have entered recovery. Reentry is often a challenge, particularly for CRNAs returning to the operating room. When we do it, we need to make sure we get it right. The authors of *Re/Entry: A Guide for Nurses Dealing With Substance Use Disorder* have done an admiral job of articulating how to do that. For their efforts, I am most grateful.

–Art Zwerling, DNP, CRNA, DAAPM

Introduction

"A journey of a thousand miles begins with a single step."

–Lao Tse

If we were sitting beside you right now, we would ask what you are seeking. So we might as well go ahead and ask: What do you want from this book? What is it you hope to find in these pages? Are you looking for information or are you looking for hope and help? Maybe both?

This book is more about direction than answers. Our belief is that by following the directions offered, you will access the answers that can make a difference in your life and the lives of others. While academic research and statistics are referenced in this book, it is not written as an academic treatise on substance use disorder (SUD) and recovery. Other writers have that angle covered. If we thought it would help you get sober, we would have quoted far more statistics. However, we never heard anyone say that what got them into treatment was hearing that overdosing on prescription meds has now surpassed car accidents as the leading cause of accidental death in the United States or how 1 out of 10 people in nursing succumb to addiction. The fact is, while statistics do tell a story, they don't get people sober. If they did, we would hand out a bunch of data and then pocket some of the billions that substance abuse costs each year while congratulating ourselves on our sobriety and superior intellect.

What does get people into treatment? Conversations, consequences, and interventions do. For this reason, we wrote this book in that order. We wrote in layers. First, we accessed our combined 35-plus years of personal recovery and decades of professional experience to write a conversation about recovery related to nursing. This book is first and foremost a conversation that we would be having if you anxiously stepped into one of our coaching sessions, called about an intervention, or showed up at a peer support group. Next, we researched academic studies. Last, we interviewed nurses in recovery and recovery professionals. Their stories and expertise are included throughout the book. This guidebook is a compilation of firsthand experience and research. It is based on our personal and professional journeys.

We are speaking to two different readers. Our predominant conversation is between someone who's been there and someone who's standing on a personal and professional precipice. We are here to share experiences, information, and stories that will give you a place to start and navigational tools for your journey. The book offers breadcrumbs leading from despair and loss back to possibility. To return is to reclaim your place as one who contributes more than you take. To return is to come out of hiding and pursue a quality life rather than squander your skills on maintaining your cover. When applied, many recovery tools can do more than restore employment. There is a great probability that you will forge a quality of life never before experienced.

Our secondary conversation is with the bystander. When you realize how close someone is to going over the edge you have two options. One is to pull out your camera phone, wonder "Will she jump?", and wait. The other is to throw her a rope. For an addict, everyone holds one end of the rope. This includes family, friends, coworkers, managers, and employers. No one knows if and when an addict will catch the rope and pull herself to safety. We don't get to decide that. The decision we have to make is whether we will be aware—ready and willing to throw the line. (Note that throwing a lifeline isn't to be confused with rescuing. More on that distinction throughout the book.)

This book offers hope and guidance for both those suffering from substance use disorder (SUD) and those standing in the emotional wake left by this disease. Both readers have something to gain from reading chapters geared toward the other. This book offers you the opportunity to lift the flap and peek inside the tent. Knowledge revealed holds the power of healing and reclamation, help for the suffering, and understanding for those watching from the sidelines. If you are standing on the outside looking in, you are far more than a spectator. Whether you are criticizing or encouraging people with addictions, jobs, lifestyles, and lives are on the line.

If you are a colleague, family member, employer, or manager of someone with SUD, it will be useful to read the whole book to know more about some of the classic mental, emotional, addictive, and circumstantial challenges encountered by nurses with SUD. You will find clarification of terms and common symptoms of addictive behavior. Beyond that, the book addresses why and how you should get involved and what is appropriate to support a nurse in recovery. You will have a clearer sense about the distinction between compassionate, clear boundaries and the ignorance of misguided judgment or enabling. One of the primary goals for this guidebook is to decrease harmful prejudice and increase a restorative culture.

Terms and Labels: What's in a Name

Because this is a guidebook, we introduce some terminology and concepts without giving you a technically thorough explanation. For that, there are volumes available in books and online. Our cursory introductions are to ensure that we're on the same page and that you know what to look up if you have more questions.

Labels are merely labels. Hopefully, in your experience, people extend beyond their labels. Obviously, labels can confirm prejudice or promote understanding. We have been very intentional about the labeling used throughout this book. While it's wieldier to write "nurse with SUD" than "impaired nurse," we are strongly opposed to that trendy term for the same reasons we do not reduce other patients to the sum total of a condition. Otherwise, we would refer to Mr. Smith as the "cancered patient in room 12." At times, it is difficult to see beyond the symptoms of any serious condition. Still, there resides a person beneath the facade. Therefore, a nurse is not an "impaired nurse." The use of *impaired* implies the nurse cannot function. Rather, the nurse may be "impaired" in any given moment while suffering from substance use disorder (SUD).

The following terms are used interchangeably throughout the book:

> *Substance use disorder (SUD)* and *addiction*
> *Drink* and *use,* both referring to ingesting or injecting a substance that creates impairment, dependency, and/or addiction

Recovery and Repetition

There is a fair amount of repetition throughout the book. The idea was not to fill more pages. Rather, this repetition exists for the following reasons:

> Some of you might not read the book cover to cover.
> A few chapters have overlapping content.
> Repetition is reinforcing. When changing perceptions, paradigms, and behaviors, repetition is key.

Repetition is vital in recovery. In early stages, it takes relentless effort to shift from compulsive behavior to liberation. Later, it takes consistency. It's like exercising. Most of us don't reach a place where we can say, "I've reached optimal health; therefore, I'm done working out." The revelation is, "It sure doesn't hurt like it did in the beginning. That part hurt. And now I feel great. I miss it when I don't work out." Recovery is the journey of a lifetime with immeasurable rewards for you and those you touch.

We are keenly grateful to all of you who are exploring recovery and shifting the addiction/recovery paradigm out of theory and into reality. As authority figures in the field of medicine, you have the opportunity to lead the way from a society blighted by addiction and its cost in lives and dollars. As you learn to identify the signs of substance abuse and offer assistance to our peers, you will also show the way for your neighbors and patients.

1

the bottom dropped out

This chapter sets the emotional stage and discusses the professional turmoil around substance abuse. Many nurses would be surprised by the number of their colleagues who have substance abuse issues. If you are one who is suffering from this, our intent is to offer you reassurance, help, and hope. As a newly recovering nurse, you will realize that you are not alone. We also intend to enlighten others about the state of mind of the nurse who is entering recovery.

Caught

You are likely reading this book for one of three reasons:

> You know or work with someone suffering from substance abuse.

> You are in trouble from substance abuse and want help.

> You have been confronted with evidence of your substance abuse.

If you are a newly recovering nurse, you may feel like the bottom has dropped out of your world. Molly felt that way.

Molly

When I was called to the office, I had an uneasy feeling. As soon as I walked in the office, I saw my handwriting—which had turned really awful—on some records my manager had printed. I had signed off on giving medicine to a patient, but she hadn't gotten it. I took it. First the manager asked me about it, and I denied any mischarting. I thought it all looked pretty genuine. Then he asked, "Are you absolutely sure there's nothing else you want to talk to me about? Or tell me?" I thought for a minute and that was my moment of clarity. I knew that I was done. I was done—confronted about all of my abuse! I said, "Yes, everything you said is true. I did it all." Then, I got walked out by management. I turned my badge in at HR where security came and got me and watched me pick up my belongings (of which I had a lot, after being there so long). Then I was escorted down to employee health, where they did the UA (tox screen). At the end, I was escorted off the premises. I had to call my mom to come pick me up because they wouldn't let me drive. That was a bad phone call. She was really angry.

After entering a program of recovery 15 years ago, Molly has reclaimed her sobriety, reclaimed herself, and recovered her family and her profession.

If you have opened this book, you are probably experiencing a variety of deep emotions such as despair, loss, humiliation, shame, remorse, resentment, and anger. Fear is the granddaddy. Categorize whatever you are experiencing as "fear." That will cover all the other emotions. Some common categories of fear include the following:

> Public humiliation
> Loss of identity and reputation
> Getting and staying clean
> Keeping or finding work
> Financial ruin
> Being outed
> Facing what you have done to patients, colleagues, your employer, and family

There might also be fear of receiving a poor employee review, losing your license, or, even worse, facing legal action, jail time, having a record, or becoming a felon.

Fear's kissing cousins are confusion and uncertainty:

> Whom do I tell? Whom don't I tell?
> Where do I begin?
> What is going to happen to me now?
> How am I going to handle this professionally, mentally, emotionally, and financially?
> I don't know who to turn to for help. Is there help?
> I feel so ashamed. I just want to hide.
> I just want to die. I could die of shame.
> This isn't me. I'm not a bad person. I'm not a person who lies, steals, and cheats, and would not want to hurt those I've been hired to care for.

> I'm a caring person and a professional caregiver.

> How did I end up violating my moral code, my professional ethics, and the laws of governance?

Maybe your response is different. Maybe you have been caught with your hand in the cookie jar and you don't know why people are making such a big deal about it. You may even boomerang between demoralization and denial. It's not uncommon to swing between these two extremes. One moment you're expressing utter despair ("I can't go on like this a minute longer!"), and a few hours later you're figuring out the quickest way to get loaded ("It's really not *that* bad!"). Denial is fueled by two agonizing consequences. First is the thought of living without your supply; it's like giving up oxygen. Then there's the unbearable thought of looking at how out of control your life has become, how far you've fallen, and how much you've betrayed those who love you.

VOICES

It's easy for denial to creep in. It causes thoughts to vacillate between extremes: "How could it have gone so wrong?" "Perhaps it's not really that bad after all. I know plenty of nurses who've taken drugs without a prescription."

If you are bound by the denial of substance abuse, there is no quality option. Your choices include the following:

> Pretending that getting high is the same thing as being happy

> Using substances to avoid feelings of despair and depression

> Avoiding thinking about how much you've lied, cheated, and stolen

> Scrambling to keep at bay consequences, such as declining health, bank account, and credibility

> Keeping yourself busy so you don't dwell on suicidal thoughts

> Realizing you can't get high anymore, but that you have to use to keep from getting sick

This is an exhausting and depressing way to live. It is also dangerous.

Join the Club

If you are experiencing degradation, denial, or both, you are far from alone. You have joined the club. This club consists of an estimated 300,000-plus nurses in the United States who are suffering from substance use disorder (SUD). That is approximately one in 10 nurses. In *Substance Use Disorder in Nursing: A Resource Manual and Guidelines for Alternative and Disciplinary Monitoring Programs* (NCSBN, 2011), the National Council of State Boards of Nursing states, "The American Nurses Association (ANA) estimates that six to eight percent of nurses use alcohol or drugs to an extent that is sufficient to impair professional performance. Others estimate that nurses generally misuse drugs and alcohol at nearly the same rate (10 to 15 percent) as the rest of the population" (p. 2). These statistics do not include nurses who have left the profession or those who have remained unidentified or unreported.

While this public-safety issue is a serious problem, there is reasonable hope for personal and professional recovery—*if* you are ready to take action and are willing to recover. This guidebook points the way to understanding and offers support for the road ahead. The requirements include the following:

> A sincere desire to recover
> Taking appropriate action guided by qualified advisors

We call these advisors your *recovery team*. Your recovery team is composed of support groups, sponsors, counselors, and monitors. If you are having surgery, you want a skilled surgeon, not a slick-talking quack. Likewise, if your life and career and sobriety are on the line, you want the right advisors. They may not say what you want to hear, but they will tell you what you need to do to stay clean.

If you merely pretend you're sincere about recovery to regain your license, you might suspend the consequences. The one guarantee, however, is that the consequences will become increasingly more grim. The three classic challenges to nurse recovery include denial of cross addiction, ego, and unresolved abuse issues. These are addressed further in later chapters.

Katie

When I first got in this program, I don't know if I was ready to quit. I had to have the want. As soon as I got the want, everything fell into place. Then I wanted to be there, I wanted to stay clean, I wanted to get through it because for a while I was like, "Just screw it. I'm just going to give up, not do anything."

The Perfect Storm: Opportunity, Motive, and Means

The phrase "perfect storm" describes the alignment of specific factors to create a catastrophic occurrence. When it comes to substance abuse, health care professionals are particularly vulnerable because the industry brings together a perfect storm of opportunity, motive, and means.

Opportunity

You already know about opportunity. Many medical treatments require pill taking and needle use as ordinary, everyday routine. It is natural to think of ingestion and injection as a reasonable response to discomfort. Combine these routines with easy access and you have opportunity. Some of the methods of opportunity are substitution, adulteration, and diversion.

> **Substitution.** Substitution is the practice of replacing one prescribed drug with another drug. It also refers to the diversion of drugs for legal and medically necessary uses to uses that are illegal and that are typically not medically authorized or necessary. For example, one nurse, Karen, recalls replacing her husband's Vicodin with Tylenol caplets. For more information, visit www.drugwarfacts.org/cms/Diversion#sthash.tVDnjyKE.dpuf.

> **Adulteration.** This refers to the alteration of any substance by the deliberate addition of a component that is not ordinarily part of that substance; typically, the substance is debased as a result (Stedman's Medical Dictionary, 2000). An example of adulteration would be siphoning off half a vial of morphine and replacing the stolen (euphemistically called "diverting") portion with saline. Many nurses—even those with SUDs—view adulteration as the worst form of tampering with patient care. It is a line that some nurses interviewed for this book thought they would never cross.

> **Diversion.** Diversion refers to the switching of drugs from legal and medically necessary uses to uses that are illegal and typically not medically authorized or necessary (Centers for Medicare & Medicaid Services, 2012). When nurses talk about diverting, they are often referring to the misappropriation of a portion of a prescribed dose for a patient. For example, a nurse might chart that Mrs. Jones took both her pain pills, when the nurse in fact gave Mrs. Jones only one and stole the second for herself. This is one of the more common ways to obtain drugs in the workplace. Skilled nursing facilities are veritable gold mines with easy opportunities to divert patient meds. One nurse, Al, recalls, "I never adulterated a vial or undermedicated a patient. I had a lot of guilt to begin with, so I didn't want to do that. I realized it was just as easy to divert to get drugs. In my 8 years of nursing, I never had another coworker or charge nurse ask to watch me waste the unused meds."

Classic methods of procurement include the following:

> Calling in prescriptions for an imaginary friend

> Requesting patients who are on narcotics

> Claiming the patient took the full dose when it was only a partial dose

Other opportunities exist, and yet more can be engineered by high-performing, high-stressed professionals pulled under by the tide of dependence.

Motive

Take a moment to reflect on personal and professional stressors. These stressors double as motives for substance abuse. One motive is the fatigue involved in working long shifts that are heavily laden with emotional and physical challenges. In addition, patients and their families are in physical and emotional pain; people in pain aren't always nice to be around. The resulting compassion fatigue along with physical strain take a hefty toll. And of course, you can only roll over so many patients or lift so many limbs for so many years before you strain your own neck, back, or arm. In addition, you have high patient acuity, too many patients, increasing workload, diminishing resources, challenging managers, and competing corporate interests, not to mention working too many nights, weekends, and holidays.

You might have personal stressors to add to the list of professional ones. Perhaps your stress got a jump start during nursing school, while you also held down a job and parented a 3-year-old. There is also a higher correlation between abuse and nurses with SUDs. Mynatt (1998) and West (2002) list family history of addictions, early victimization—particularly verbal, physical, and sexual abuse—and the experience of losing a loved one as early risk factors for SUDs.

Jamie

There was a class I took in treatment called "Seeking Safety," basically about PTSD and addiction. It listed some of the qualifiers: high stress job, trauma, childhood trauma, lots of different criteria. Out of the list of 12 items, I had 11!

I looked at the patterns in my life and thought, "Oh my God!" It was a process of recognition of some of my childhood traumas, some marital traumas, and the choices I had made. I had wanted to get back into an ER position but then I thought, "Oh, that will just feed my disease." I know if I go back into trauma right now my addiction could flare up again and I'm not going there. So it was a blessing I didn't get an ER job.

Means

Physical and emotional motives are shored up by the means. In the nursing context, this can be ignorance combined with some general characteristics associated with people in the helping professions. Regarding the latter, how well-equipped do you feel to deal with patients suffering from effects of substance abuse (beyond treating the immediate symptoms)? Take it one step further. How much time did your nursing education devote to the professional liability for SUDs? One three-credit course? A chapter? A role-play? Or less? Did your professor point out that one in 10 of you were statistically vulnerable? Then did you discuss how to look for your own warning signs? Did you role-play what to look for and how to respond to a coworker suffering from SUDs? Imagine avoiding the topic of crash-landing a plane in flight school.

The personality tendencies of service providers escalate the means. As an exercise, write down some of the tendencies and personality traits of people drawn to helping professions such as nursing:

_____

_____

_____

_____

_____

While there surely are differences in individuals, we're guessing at least some of the following traits crossed your mind: nurturer, caretaker, high achiever, altruist, codependent, detail-oriented, good in a crisis, trauma/chaos/ adrenaline junkie. Often, helpers leave themselves out of the equation. (See Appendix D, "Circle of Care.") Because they find it hard to help them-selves, they rationalize: "I will take a pill rather than take a stand, change lifestyle habits, learn stress-reduction techniques, or talk to a counselor."

Although it has become more common for people to talk about having healthy boundaries, implementing responsible self-care may require relative-ly new behaviors for some nurses. This can be an even greater feat for people who have suffered boundary violations as children. Combine flimsy bound-aries with the impulse of many in helping professions to focus on the needs of others, and the stage is set for experiencing more mental, emotional, and physical pain than is healthy. Sublimating personal welfare and tolerating increasing levels of discomfort create more susceptibility to substance abuse. Often, the more people shortcut their well-being, the more shortcuts are re-quired later to get by—such as diverting a patient's pain meds to get through the workday. Combine genetic predisposition, easy access, and multiple stressors with a mindset that melds comfort and confidence in drug use, and you have a slippery slide from use to abuse. You are trapped inside the per-fect storm.

VOICES

If you could read minds, you might overhear a nurse thinking, "I am on my third 12-hour shift in a row, with a strained back and a heavy patient load. My kid kept me awake all night, and I feel a headache coming on. I can just take that extra pill my patient declined. That will get me through."

While your personal nightmare, career status, and monitoring requirements may appear daunting, there is reason for hope. There is no known cure for SUDs, but if you are ready for healing, there is a road to recovery—and a life of recovery can be filled with joy and purpose. How far you take the road is up to you and no one but you. The potential for healing, deeper self-awareness, greater capacity to serve, and freedom from old ghosts are some of the side effects of a life of recovery. This guidebook is here to calm your fears, inform you of the help available, and discuss some of the challenges ahead. It might look like a steep climb, but the view from the top makes it worth moving through the fear of heights, bloody noses, and sweaty tears. Unlike the dulled pain and despair of substance abuse, recovery is pain with a purpose.

Brent's Story

I went to the board of nursing to renew my dues for my nursing license. The board members asked, "Okay what's going on?" They saw that I had had two DUIs in Denver. I had been sober 90 days at that point and, after treatment, was all fired up about honesty and openness. So I shared my history with them.

This is my story: I had been drinking heavily, and I had been missing work. It hadn't gotten to a point where the manager was ready to let me go. She knew that I had been missing work and often looked hung over. But she could tell something was going on in my life. I wasn't always "Brent." My manager, my mentor, had hired me, and she cared. She said, "Brent, you're keeping it together. You're a great person, but you have issues right now." She knew that I had gone to EAP. So I quit my job and did a geographic to Denver. I thought my life would change with new friends and new scenery, but it got a lot worse. I got two DUIs and still continued heavy drinking.

My brother and a former sister-in-law lived in Denver, but I isolated myself from them because I didn't want them to see me. For a month and a half, I continued to go down to the bottom. I was from a good background. I had a great job. I was a professional, but there I was in an empty house, I didn't shower, didn't eat. My house was horrible. My poor dog. All I had were cushions on the floor in my bedroom, my dog, and a TV. I couldn't get in the car to drive because I couldn't stop abusing sleeping pills and booze.

My mother called one morning and asked, "Are you okay?" because she hadn't heard from me. She kept calling and I'd say, "I'm going to be there in a couple of days." After the third phone call, because she was so worried, I said, "I need help." My brother came immediately. He saw the condition I was in. He took care of some affairs, threw me in a car with my dog, and drove me to my hometown. Four days later, I was in Pine Grove, rehab program. I was there for 90 days.

Later, after a month of being back home, being sober, and going to 90 in 90 (90 meetings in 90 days), I went to the board of nursing to get my license back because I was broke. My parents were supporting me. I remember thinking, "I'm sober. I feel better. I'm fine, I'm okay." And I was invited by the board to sign a contract for 3 years.

I was angry at myself for a while, but I look back now and say, the best thing that ever happened to me was getting into that program for 3 years. It brought things forward that I hadn't been honest about—my drinking, the unmanageability. It gave me discipline: discipline to avoid self-medicating because of the random UAs. I was responsible for being on time to required meetings. The program compelled me to get to more AA meetings than I would have on my own. It also allowed me to continue to work and be in my chosen profession. Nursing was part of me. I had been a nurse for over 9 years when I signed my contract.

I interviewed at a hospital and got hired. I had known the clinical supervisor on that floor. I knew a few other people there. They said, "He's a great nurse; we want him." So when I came back in for the second interview and was offered the job, I said, "Okay, time out. Thank you, but I need to tell you something first." I told the supervisor that I was in the PRN program. I showed her the requirements; she would have to report to the program monitor on a quarterly basis how I was doing. She said, "I have absolutely no problem whatsoever; I've done this before." They checked my references. They knew how I lost my job in Denver. She said, "Here you go, let's go." And I said, "Thank you!"

One thing I admired was the confidentiality that my manager offered. Her integrity was incredible. She let me tell my own story, and I respected that. She offered open arms and trust, giving me a chance without judgment. I never had a feeling like I was being watched over, even from the people I opened up to. I worked for that fabulous manager for 6 years. I was always on time and went 2 years without an absence. I was "on time reliable."

There is a silence in our society. There is a silence in nursing. When I was in school for my bachelor's, SUD was never discussed. I would love to see it discussed and maybe combined with a lecture on civility. Some of the students in my classes thought that the civility topic was needed in the first semester to know how to deal with classmates, instructors, administrators, and staff teaching clinicals. I think they could be put together—civility with the substance abuse issue.

When speaking of silence, I wasn't comfortable in our society. I had always been under the radar because I didn't feel safe disclosing my sexuality. A lot of that carried over from my childhood until I got sober. Carrying the secret of being gay was some of my emotional buildup, but it was not a cause of my addiction.

I think our society has come around a lot to accept that people who are in sobriety can return to work. I was lucky because some hospitals are not accepting of people with the disease of substance use disorder.

When I first got into AA, I was complaining about an ankle bracelet for home detention because of my DUI. I harped to a person of substantial sobriety, "God, I gotta do this, I gotta do that, I gotta go to this meeting, I gotta get a UA, I got this ankle bracelet and it hurts. Waaah." He turned around and said, "Just stop it right there. I have to ask you one question. Did you invite these people into your life?" And I had to say yes. That was a turning point for me. Okay, you've invited this into your life—these people, this sanction. In the beginning, I looked at it as punishment. But it's not punishment. You invited them. If you take advantage of recovery, it's a good thing.

Recovery, to say the very least, has saved my life. I am employable, reliable, a good friend, and a good brother. Before my parents died, I became a good son. That felt good, especially since they helped me get sober. I truly believe I would be dead without the support of the fellowship (AA). The support of family and friends and the PRN program were all essential to my recovery. They gave me discipline and accountability, also allowing me to work and support myself while beginning the journey of living sober. I truly believe that PRN was the best thing that happened in my recovery. What a gift!

At first, faith was difficult for me. Now, evidence that God works in my life every day is one of the biggest gifts of all. If my story reaches others on this earth and helps another person choose recovery, I will be fulfilled.

Today I can achieve and reach for anything, only because I am sober and living in recovery! Thank God for AA! I'm just so darned grateful and happy for the kind of life I have now!

References

Adulteration. (2000). In *Stedman's Medical Dictionary* (26th ed.). Philadelphia, PA: Lippincott Williams & Wilkins. Retrieved from http://www.drugs.com/dict/adulteration.html

Centers for Medicare & Medicaid Services. (2012). Drug diversion in the Medicaid program: State strategies for reducing prescription drug diversion in Medicaid. Baltimore, MD: Centers for Medicare & Medicaid Services, p. 1. Retrieved from http://www.drugwarfacts.org/cms/Diversion#sthash.tVDnjyKE.FXqqTH26.dpuf

Mynatt, S.L. (1998). Increasing resiliency to substance abuse in recovering women with comorbid depression. *Journal of Psychosocial Nursing, 3*(1), 28–36.

National Council of State Boards of Nursing, Substance Use Disorder Committee. (2011). Substance use disorder in nursing. Retrieved from https://www.ncsbn.org/SUDN_10.pdf

Reference.MD. (n.d.). Drug substitution. *Reference.MD.* Retrieved from http://www.reference.md/files/D057/mD057915.html

West, M. (2002). Early risk indicators of substance abuse among nurses. *Journal of Nursing Scholarship, 34*(2), 187–193.

2

overview of addiction and recovery: setting the stage

We believe those who can heal themselves through surrender, dedication, and support in turn become the real healers of the world. Much of healing depends on understanding and communication. This chapter provides a cultural context for general concepts and terms related to drug/alcohol abuse, dependency, and recovery. Included are descriptions of common defense mechanisms and areas of denial.

Joining the Club

As mentioned in Chapter 1, "The Bottom Dropped Out," opening this book establishes your membership into a club that has members with substance use disorder (SUD) issues. Affiliate members know someone with SUD issues. Most everyone in the United States is an affiliate member of this club, whether they know it or not. Following are some national statistics that bear witness:

> In 2011, an estimated 2.5 million Americans aged 12 or older were illicit drug users. Slightly more than half (51.8 percent) of Americans aged 12 or older reported being current drinkers of alcohol. This translates to an estimated 133.4 million current drinkers, according to Substance Abuse and Mental Health Services Administration (SAMHSA, 2011, p. 31). "The Office of National Drug Control Policy lists the second most frequent illicit drug abuse problem as the abuse of prescription medication. This problem affects 48 million, or 20 percent, of Americans aged 12 and older each year...Drug Abuse Warning Network (DAWN) reports that benzodiazepines and opioid pain relievers are responsible for large increases—170 percent and 450 percent, respectively—in the number of visits to emergency rooms" (Baird, 2011, p. 72).

> Nearly two-thirds of American families have direct experience with alcohol or drug addiction (Hart, 2004). Statistics alone support the need for greater awareness and guidelines for responding to SUDs. This disease affects quality of life and financially strains our society.

> In California alone, it has been estimated that problems related to alcohol consumption cost approximately $38.5 billion in health services, work losses, criminal-justice spending, property damage, and costs of public programs (Rosen, Miller, & Simon, 2008).

> Drug abuse costs the United States' economy hundreds of billions of dollars in increased health care costs, increased crime, and lost productivity. The total costs of drug abuse and addiction due to use of tobacco, alcohol, and illegal drugs are estimated at $524 billion each year. Illicit drug use alone accounts for $181 billion in health care, productivity loss, crime, incarceration, and drug enforcement (National Institute on Drug Abuse, 2010).

> SUD statistics for nurses are commensurate with national statistics. However, while overall substance use rates in nursing are comparable to the general population, nurses are more likely to abuse prescription-type drugs than the overall population (NCSBN, 2011).

Statistics support one reason for treating SUDs: Treatment services pay for themselves (Ettner, Huang, Evans, Ash, Hardy, Jourabchi, & Hser, 2006; Wickizer, Krupski, Stark, Mancuso, & Campbell, 2006). In fact, SUD treatment in Washington state was determined to net a cost savings of approximately $2,500 annually per person, a figure that approximated the cost of an episode of substance-abuse treatment during that period (Wickizer et al., 2006).

Defining Recovery

Because recovery is the heart of this book, it is ironic that it is one of the most elusive terms to define. There is no universally accepted definition of recovery. It lives more as a description than a definition. More than a static state or a fixed point in a destination, recovery refers to personal development and a lifestyle and that includes outlook, abstinence, liberation from your compulsion, and a return to more mental, physical, and emotional well-being.

For a person with a substance use disorder, *recovery* is the process of getting well. Getting well does not mean finding a cure, but it does mean regaining control of one's life. It is marked by the individual's acceptance of having a substance use disorder and abstaining from alcohol and all unauthorized, nonprescribed drugs (National Council of State Boards of Nursing, 2011). Another definition of recovery is from John Kleinig (2008, p. 1702): "A process or outcome in which a disabling burden is overcome and an affirmative state of being or wellness is established."

Often, people who have successfully overcome their dependence on alcohol and other drugs describe themselves as being "in recovery." This is consistent with the working definition of recovery put forth by a panel of experts convened by the Betty Ford Institute: "a voluntarily maintained lifestyle characterized by sobriety, personal health, and citizenship." The panel also noted, "Recovery may be the best word to summarize all the positive benefits to physical, mental, and social health that can happen when alcohol- and other drug-dependent individuals get the help they need" (The Betty Ford Institute Consensus Panel, 2007, p. 225).

It is important to note that while complete abstinence from alcohol and all other nonprescribed drugs is a necessary component of recovery, abstinence alone does not equate to a lifestyle of recovery. The panel listed what they consider to be three levels of sobriety that indicate movement toward a recovery lifestyle.

> **Early.** Between 1 and 12 months of abstinence
> **Sustained.** Between 1 and 5 years of abstinence
> **Stable.** More than 5 years of sobriety

Individuals deemed "stable" are said to be at lower risk of relapse.

NOTE | *Because the recovery tools and principles are the same for alcohol and all other drugs, we use the terms drink and use, alcohol and drugs, and alcoholic and addict interchangeably. For example, if we wrote, "I quit using," you can mentally replace it with "I quit drinking."*

NOTE *There is no known cure for the disease of addiction. However, just as a diabetic is always a diabetic, he or she can choose a path to well-being.*

Here, we encourage you to remember what being healthy felt like. Many people suffering from SUD have reclaimed and even transcended their previous quality of life. The result is that they experience more joy, community, and peace after a consistent and persistent period of recovery. However, for you right now, feeling well may seem impossible or something from a foreign land. Persist, and things will shift.

Dr. Nora Volkow, director at National Institute on Drug Abuse (NIDA), has been instrumental in demonstrating that drug addiction is a disease of the human brain. The big news that Volkow has found is that most addicts share a reduction in levels of dopamine receptors. This isn't just for the hard drugs; this includes people who regularly smoke marijuana and cigarettes. The brain isn't wired to handle these highs, and a shut-off valve kicks in and reduces the number of receptors available. So the ability of the drugs to stimulate pleasure continues to decrease. That is why eventually addicts no longer use to get high, but just to feel normal. On top of that, drugs have been shown to damage the prefrontal cortex; this is the area that resides in the front of the brain and is the executive function that allows us to exert free will. When this is damaged, it makes it more difficult to regulate emotions and self-control (Goldstein, 2012).

In recovery, you will struggle to deal with damage done not only to your brain, but to relationships, finances, and health, as well as other areas. You can expect relief to come in intervals, and can expect these states of ease to be interrupted by times of fear, pain, and—most dangerously—denial. After the physical cravings have subsided, it is typical to get discouraged and feel like you're never going to climb out of this hole. "I might as well be using," you might say. "At least then I don't have to feel like this anymore." That translates to, "I don't want to deal with all the fear, pain, and anxiety." It is easy to relapse.

A recovery program is the most effective antidote to mental/emotional re-lapse. Tools and support groups are powerful countermeasures for isolation, negative thinking, and destructive behaviors. The only requisite is genuine dedication to active recovery. In this regard, recovery is more than an idea. It is a program of action you take with others—a sponsor, counselor, coach, and/or support group(s).

To recover from the use and preoccupation with substances of any kind, you must use the tools of recovery. Just as you do not expect to see physi-cal changes without doing something different, nor enjoy a book without reading it, without action you cannot reap the benefits that accompany a recovery program.

Classic Traps and Defense Mechanisms

One way to avoid true recovery is to pretend you have embraced a healthy program. In the language of recovery, this is called *fronting*. Fronting is go-ing through the motions to manipulate others into thinking that all is well. You say and appear to do the right things, but you only act this way so that you can use later when no one is paying attention. Fronting is work-ing the system instead of changing internally. Fronting is a huge challenge to people who monitor and treat SUDs. It is difficult to tell if people are sincere about their recovery based on their words or demeanor. You might be genuinely in recovery or fronting recovery. This book is not written, nor will it be effective, for those who wish to front recovery to reclaim a good image or paycheck.

From Fronting to Denial

Sometimes you're so convincing that you start believing your own fabrica-tions. You begin to forget when you're lying because you've been selling the story for so long. If you are an addicted nurse, there was likely some point where you began to think it was acceptable to justify diverting drugs from a patient. To an addict, it feels like doing what you need to do to survive, just like you're driven to get food even if it means stealing. The drive to feed the hunger of addiction feels as innate as the drive to eat and drink.

Classic traps for relapse include the following:

> Denial

> Isolation

> Staying with using friends

> Changing too much at once or not changing anything

> Self-sponsorship or "working your own program"

> Resisting help, instruction, and guidance

NOTE | *One of the classic relapse traps is denial, which is a defense mechanism.*

Nurses study defense mechanisms in school, so they are familiar with the topic. An interpretation was given by Grohol (2007, p. 1): "Defense mechanisms are one way of looking at how people distance themselves from a full awareness of unpleasant thoughts, feelings, and behaviors." The following are definitions of some major defense mechanisms:

> **Denial.** As noted by Grohol (2007, p. 4), "Denial is the refusal to accept reality or fact, acting as if a painful event, thought, or feeling did not exist. It is considered one of the most primitive of the defense mechanisms because it is characteristic of early childhood development. Many people use denial in their everyday lives to avoid dealing with painful feelings or areas of their life they don't wish to admit. For instance, a person who is a functioning alcoholic will often simply deny she has a drinking problem, pointing to how well she functions in her job and relationships."

> **Compartmentalization.** This lesser form of dissociation means parts of oneself are separated from awareness of other parts and behaving as if one has separate sets of values. An example is an honest person who cheats on his or her income tax return, keeping the two value systems distinct and unintegrated while remaining unconscious of the cognitive dissonance.

> **Projection.** The misattribution of a person's undesired thoughts, feelings, or impulses onto another person who does not have those thoughts, feelings, or impulses is projection (Grohol, 2007). Projection is used especially when the thoughts are considered unacceptable for the person to express or the person feels completely ill at ease having them. For example, a person may be angry at his or her spouse for not listening, when in fact it is the angry spouse who does not listen. Projection is often the result of a lack of insight and acknowledgment of one's own motivations and feelings.

> **Rationalization.** Rationalization is putting something into a different light or offering a different explanation for one's perceptions or behaviors in the face of a changing reality (Grohol, 2007). For instance, suppose a woman who starts dating a man she really, really likes and thinks the world of is suddenly dumped by the man for no reason. She might reframe the situation in her mind by thinking, "I suspected he was a loser all along."

> **Minimization.** Cognitive distortion can result in minimization (Grohol, 2007). When people are thinking with the cognitive distortion of magnification and minimization, they are either blowing things out of proportion or lessening their importance (Star, 2011).

> **Isolation.** While isolation is not identified as a defense mechanism, it is a dominant tendency for addicts. Addiction has been referred to as a disease of isolation. Isolation becomes necessary to prevent others from seeing the increasing level of substance abuse by the addict. This is usually accompanied by a decrease in social engagement. It is ironic that people who started out drinking or using to loosen up and feel more "normal" revert to even greater antisocial tendencies as the disorder progresses (Myers, 2002).

> **Justification.** Someone can attempt to justify behavior or vindicate oneself. Justification is an attempt to relieve the user of blame. ("You'd drink too if you were married to my husband, had to raise my kids, and had to work for my boss.")

Common Addiction Terminology

Labels are labels. They can be limiting and prejudicial, or helpful and revealing. Therefore, we have been very intentional about the wording used throughout this book. In this and subsequent chapters, *substance use disorder (SUD)* is used interchangeably with *impaired/impairment* and *addicted/addiction*. We opted not to use the phrase *impaired nurse(s)* for the following reason:

> The term "impaired" is specifically not used because a person with a substance use disorder is not necessarily impaired; that is, always functioning poorly or incompetently. On the contrary, a nurse with a substance use disorder can be high-functioning and high-achieving. It's a myth that all alcoholics are skid row drunks and that all those with a substance use disorder are necessarily impaired (National Council of State Boards of Nursing, 2011, p. 3).

In addition, we view each individual as a person first, rather than an addict with a disease that has debilitating symptoms. The person is not defective or impaired, but when active in the disorder, he or she *becomes* impaired. Even the designation of state programs is based on the old punishment model—punitive/dismissal and alternative-to-discipline program. That description is counter to this book's intentions. Therapeutic nomenclature— that is, *restorative nurse program* or *program for recovering nurses (PRN)*—serves the intention more accurately.

All that being said, people do need to speak a common language when talking about substance abuse. In discussing recovery, some common conceptions and misconceptions are related to the language. This section defines common terms used when dealing with addiction and recovery. It also delves into common recovery vernacular, many of which are taken from Alcoholics Anonymous (AA) and Narcotics Anonymous (NA) literature. (You learn can more about AA and NA in Chapter 4, "Treatment Options.")

> **Addiction:** A primary, chronic, neurobiological disease, with genetic, psychosocial, and environmental factors influencing its development and manifestations. It is characterized by behaviors that include one or more of the following: impaired control over drug use, compulsive use, continued use despite harm, and craving (National Institute on Drug Abuse). There is also the American Society of Addiction Medicine's (ASAM, 2011, p. 1) new definition of addiction:

> Addiction is a primary, chronic disease of brain reward, motivation, memory, and related circuitry. Addiction affects neurotransmission and interactions within reward structures of the brain, including the nucleus accumbens, anterior cingulate cortex, basal forebrain and amygdala, such that motivational hierarchies are altered and addictive behaviors, which may or may not include alcohol and other drug use, supplant healthy, self care-related behaviors. Addiction also affects neurotransmission and interactions between cortical and hippocampal circuits and brain reward structures, such that the memory of previous exposures to rewards (such as food, sex, alcohol, and other drugs) leads to a biological and behavioral response to external cues, in turn triggering craving and/or engagement in addictive behaviors.

> **Alcoholism:** A primary, chronic disease with genetic, psychosocial, and environmental factors influencing its development and manifestations. The disease is often progressive and fatal. It is characterized by

continuous or periodic impaired control over drinking, preoccupation with the drug alcohol, use of alcohol despite adverse consequences, and distortions in thinking, most notably denial (American Society of Addiction Medicine, 1990).

> **Chemical dependency:** A medical disorder in which an individual experiences a compulsion to take a drug, either continuously or periodically, to experience its psychic effects or to avoid the discomfort of its absence (National Council of State Boards of Nursing, 2011, p. 236).

> **Craving:** The urge for drugs after ceasing drug use. Craving is both a physiological response as well as a conditioned response to people, places, and things previously associated with drug use (National Council of State Boards of Nursing, 2011, p. 236).

> **Dependence:** Includes such symptoms as drug taking in larger amounts than intended, inability to cut down on drug use, a great deal of time spent in activities necessary to obtain the drug, and continued use despite knowledge of health or social problems caused by the drug. Dependence may or may not include physical dependence, which, according to NIDA (Gaufberg, Barnes, Albanese & Cohen, 2009, p. 6), is defined as "a state of adaptation that is manifested by a drug class-specific withdrawal syndrome that can be produced by abrupt cessation, rapid dose reduction, decreasing blood level of the drug, and/or administration of an antagonist." The Diagnostic and Statistical Manual of Mental Disorders IV (DSM-IV) term *dependence* is what NIDA refers to as *addiction*.

> **Drug addiction (substance use disorder):** A chronic relapsing brain disorder characterized by neurobiological changes that lead to a compulsion to take a drug with loss of control over drug intake. It is characterized by the compulsive use of drugs and the inability to stop using them despite all the problems caused by their use. A person with an addiction is unable to stop the behavior, be it drinking or taking drugs or something else, despite serious health, economic, vocational, legal, spiritual, and social consequences (National Council of State Boards of Nursing, 2011, p. 236).

Those who are dependent are losing themselves to the drug. The old saying is, "The man takes a drink, then the drink takes a drink, then the drink takes the man." And the difference between good and GOOD is the biochemical differences that occur in my head when I drink versus when somebody else drinks, and to me that's the powerlessness of the disease; I can't change that. I cannot change what happens to my central nervous system when the alcohol hits it. The only thing I can change is whether or not I imbibe the alcohol. So yes, at some point I do have choices. When I'm in the middle of it, I don't have a choice, because it's doing what it does, and what it does is the drink is taking a drink, and that's not something that happens to normies. When you're thirsty and you drink, you get full. When I'm thirsty and I drink, I get more thirsty.

–Mark H. Broadhead, MD

- **Drug diversion:** A variety of activities used to obtain drugs illegally. It is most commonly used to refer to the misappropriation of drugs from a patient, health care employer, or other source (National Council of State Boards of Nursing, 2011, p. 236).

- **Dual diagnosis:** Co-occurrence of a mental illness, drug addiction, and/or alcoholism in various combinations.

- **Impairment:** In this context, functioning poorly or incompetently due to substance abuse.

- **Recovery:** As defined at the beginning of this chapter, the process for a person with an SUD to achieve well-being.

- **Relapse:** The return to drug or alcohol use after a period of abstinence. A relapse may last for a few days or for many years. Relapse is not a simple, singular event; rather, it is a long process that usually begins with distancing oneself from participation in meetings and results in the reemergence of denial. A person loses sight of the benefits of recovery and becomes reabsorbed in his or her addictive substance (National Council of State Boards of Nursing, 2011, p. 238).

> **Sobriety:** The state of abstinence from mind-altering drugs and alcohol. However, not everyone who is abstinent will achieve sobriety. Sobriety describes people who are striving to find a balanced life that includes a holistic approach to recovery. It involves the health of the mind, body, and spirit.

> **Substance abuse:** Any use of drugs in a manner deviating from medically approved or socially acceptable patterns either on a single occasion or episodically. For example, a nurse who uses on duty on one occasion is exhibiting poor judgment and putting clients at risk but is not necessarily addicted (National Council of State Boards of Nursing, 2011, p. 239).

> **Substance use disorder (SUD):** A maladaptive pattern of substance use leading to clinically significant impairment or distress, as manifested by two or more of the following occurring within a 12-month period (DSM-V):

>> Recurrent substance use resulting in a failure to fulfill major role obligations at work, school, or home (for example, repeated absences or poor work performance related to substance use)

>> Substance-related absences, suspensions, or expulsions from school

>> Neglect of children or household

>> Recurrent substance use in situations where it is physically hazardous (for example, driving an automobile or operating a machine when impaired)

>> Continued substance use despite having persistent or recurrent social or interpersonal problems caused or exacerbated by the effects of the substance (for example, arguments with spouse about consequences of intoxication, physical fights)

> **Tolerance:** The phenomenon of needing to use larger amounts of drugs to attain the same effect of a non-user using a much smaller amount of the drug (National Council of State Boards of Nursing, 2011, p. 239).

> **Withdrawal:** The group of symptoms that occurs upon the abrupt discontinuation or decrease in intake of medications or recreational drugs. Withdrawal symptoms can range from mild to severe intensity with dangerous complications.

Recovery Program Terminology

Here are common terms you will encounter in support groups and treatment programs. Many of them come from the archetypical recovery programs Alcoholics Anonymous (AA) and Narcotics Anonymous (NA).

> **90 in 90 (AA/NA):** Suggestion that newcomers attend 90 meetings in 90 days. If missing a day is unavoidable, you can double or triple up meetings on other days. The purpose is to assist a newcomer to prevent relapse and promote a pattern of recovery during a significantly vulnerable phase.

> **AA's primary purpose:** To stay sober and help other alcoholics achieve sobriety.

> **Abstinence:** Not drinking alcohol at all. Abstinence, AA believes, is the only treatment for the disease of alcoholism.

> **Acceptance:** One of AA's primary principles to accept the things in life that cannot be changed, including the disease of alcoholism and the inability to drink normally. *See* Serenity Prayer.

> **Alcoholism (described by AA):** While there is no medical definition of alcoholism used in AA/NA, many describe it as a physical compulsion coupled with a mental obsession. In other words, an alcoholic has a distinct physical desire to consume alcohol beyond his or her capacity to control it and in defiance of all commonsense rules. Not only do alcoholics have an abnormal craving for alcohol, but they frequently yield to it at the worst possible times. They do not know when or how to stop drinking.

> **Big Book:** The nickname given to the book *Alcoholics Anonymous*, so named because of the unusual thickness of the paper on which it was

originally printed. Although the book is now smaller, the nickname stuck and is, in fact, registered.

> **Break anonymity:** To reveal one's own or someone else's membership in AA or to repeat something that was said by someone in an AA meeting. There are only four reasons for breaking anonymity at a personal level:

> > It will help you stay sober.

> > It will help someone else stay sober.

> > People in your life need to know.

> > It will prevent you from having to lie.

> **Clean:** A state of abstinence, free of inappropriate substance. This term can indicate a clear urinalysis but not necessarily a program of good recovery.

> **Codependent:** Coined originally to describe the relationship between an alcoholic and his or her partner. Now used more generally to describe enabling actions, a lack of self-esteem, and an unhealthy need to fix another person, thereby abandoning one's own needs and identity.

> **Contempt prior to investigation:** This phrase appears in a quotation of Herbert Spencer's, found in Appendix II of the Big Book: "There is a principle which is a bar against all information, which is proof against all arguments and which cannot fail to keep a man in everlasting ignorance—that principle is contempt prior to investigation." The phase is often used as a warning against being closed to new ideas. Open-mindedness is an essential part of recovery.

> **Dry:** Being abstinent from alcohol. To those in AA, however, being dry is just one small part of being sober. Sobriety is a way of life based on spiritual principles. To remain dry without changing intellectually, emotionally, and spiritually is to be dangerously close to the next drink. The Big Book (Alcoholics Anonymous, 2013, p. 31) says, "We feel that elimination of our drinking is but a beginning."

> **Dry drunk:** A condition of returning to one's old alcoholic thinking and behavior without actually drinking. Also known as *dry bender.*

> **Enabling:** A term used to describe overly compassionate behavior toward an alcoholic. This works against a drinking alcoholic's recovery because it keeps him or her from having to deal with the consequences of his or her behavior. Examples of enabling are making excuses for the alcoholic and cleaning up after one of his or her "episodes." The alcoholic needs to face all the unpleasant consequences of drinking if he or she is to recover.

> **Geographical cure:** While still drinking, an effort to cure alcoholism by getting a "fresh start" in a new location. It doesn't work. There is a saying around AA: "Wherever you go, there you are." Also known as *geographic* or *pulling a geographic.*

> **H.A.L.T.:** An acronym for "hungry, angry, lonely, or tired." It is in these states when resolve is the weakest. The acronym reminds addicts to always try to avoid or repair these states in an effort to protect their recovery.

> **Higher power:** A self-defined power greater than oneself to which one ultimately turns for assistance and guidance in one's sober life. In an alcoholic's drinking days, alcohol is the higher power. In sobriety, you choose a different kind of power to fulfill your purpose. Because AA is nonsectarian, the definition of higher power is left entirely to the individual.

> **Hitting bottom:** Reaching such a state of utter hopelessness that one becomes willing to admit complete defeat in dealing with one's alcoholism. In such a state, the alcoholic becomes "teachable" and is willing to do whatever is necessary to achieve sobriety. The bottom the alcoholic hits at the end of his or her drinking days is usually emotional and spiritual. It may or may not involve other complications such as poor health, financial problems, and legal problems.

> **Insanity:** AA's (2013, p. 25) second step states, "We came to believe that a power greater than ourselves could restore us to sanity." Some-

times, AA members hear insanity defined as "doing the same thing over and over but expecting different results."

> **Intervention:** The process by which family members and/or friends of an alcoholic join together and confront the alcoholic about the negative effects of his or her behavior. The goal of an intervention is to break through the alcoholic's denial of his or her problem and to motivate the alcoholic to seek help. Intervention is often a means of assisting an alcoholic to hit his or her bottom long before he or she would naturally.

> **One day at a time:** This slogan describes one of AA's primary strategies for staying sober. For many alcoholics, the concept of permanent abstinence is too overwhelming. Most, however, believe they can stay sober for a 24-hour period. If an AA member feels he or she absolutely, positively must have a drink, he or she puts it off until tomorrow or until the next 15 minutes, if necessary. This gives the member time to call his or her sponsor, get to a meeting, or pray to his or her higher power to remove the craving.

> **Principles before personalities:** This phrase comes from the 12th AA (2013, ¶ 75) tradition, "Anonymity is the spiritual foundation of all our traditions, ever reminding us to place principles before personalities." It is the principles of the program, rather than personalities, that guide recovery and keep us sober. We rely on the 12 steps and their principles rather than on one individual or group of individuals. Individuals, regardless of how charismatic, are only human. Our ultimate reliance is on our higher power.

> **Resentment:** Feelings of ill will that we hold for others, usually as a result of some perceived harm they have done us. In recovery, one cannot afford to harbor resentments. They corrode one's life and "justified" resentments can lead one back to relapse. The Big Book (A.A., 2013, p. 66) says, "It is plain that a life which includes deep resentment leads only to futility and unhappiness. To the precise extent that we permit these, do we squander the hours that might have been worthwhile."

> **Rigorous honesty:** Chapter 5 in the Big Book (A.A., n.d., p. 58) asserts that addicts who do not recover "are naturally incapable of grasping and developing a manner of living which demands rigorous honesty." Rigorous honesty is characterized by the complete lack of intent to deceive one's self or anyone else.

> **Serenity Prayer:** Reinhold Niebuhr's Serenity Prayer reads, in part, "God, grant me the serenity to accept the things I cannot change, the courage to change the things I can, and wisdom to know the difference." This prayer is often used as a mantra of sorts by AA members. It is a powerful tool for achieving balance when emotions threaten to overwhelm.

> **Slip:** A controversial term for relapse, or drinking alcohol again after a period of sobriety. The term is used as an acronym for *sobriety loses its priority*. Addiction professionals are apt to consider a slip as different from a relapse in intent and duration, where 12-step culture can view the term *slip* as minimizing the danger of any form of relapse.

> **Sponsor:** For those who are fond of acronyms, S.P.O.N.S.O.R. stands for *sober person offering a newcomer suggestions on recovery*. A sponsor is an AA member who serves as a mentor of sorts to a newcomer in the program. A sponsor typically helps a sponsee to work the 12 steps; shares his or her personal experience, strength, and hope; and helps the sponsee stay on the recovery track. Although not mentioned in the Big Book, sponsorship has become widely accepted as a crucial part of the recovery program.

> **Stinking thinking:** This phrase refers to an alcoholic's reversion to old thought patterns and attitudes. Stinking thinking may include blaming others, grandiosity, fault-finding, self-centeredness, and skipping meetings. This kind of thinking warns an alcoholic that he or she is not working the AA program and is getting precariously close to the next drink.

> **Surrender:** To surrender in AA is to effectively take the first three steps, summarized as: 1) admitting that we are powerless over alcohol

and that our lives have become unmanageable, 2) coming to believe that a power greater than ourselves could restore us to sanity, and 3) turning our will and our lives over to the care of God as we understand Him. Surrender is the key to recovery. Only when an addict completely surrenders is he or she willing to let a power greater than himself or herself restore sanity.

> **Terminally unique:** An alcoholic's idea that his or her uniqueness exempts him or her from some part of the AA program or the 12 steps. AA does not deny that each individual is a unique creation. However, as alcoholics, we have far more similarities than we have differences. There is an expression in AA literature: "Always remember that you are unique, just like everyone else."

> **Tools:** The expression "Use your tools" refers to all devices and actions that support recovery, such as working steps with a sponsor, using new mantras, pausing when agitated, and thinking things through. Part of a recovery team's job is to introduce these tools.

> **Working the program:** Attending meetings faithfully, reading AA literature regularly, applying what you learn to daily living, sharing with others, and accepting with an open mind what they share.

> **Working the steps:** Commencing and continuing the 12-step course of action prescribed by AA for recovery. It is best undertaken with the guidance of a sponsor

Gabe's Story

Sweet relief...eventually!

Ever since I was in high school, I found the idea of altering how I felt interesting. I had no reason to think other people did not also feel this way. After high school, I went into the Marine Corps. Compliance in the military was mandatory. I did not come close to using any drugs. I remember a fellow Marine losing rank because he smoked pot. "Not me! Never!" I thought to myself.

After getting out of the service, I went to college, eventually making my way to becoming an RN. Through the years leading up to finishing my RN degree, I started using alcohol to change the way I felt. I thought my life was not progressing as envisioned, that I was not becoming the person I was supposed to be. I wasn't married and was generally discontent. Alcohol seemed to help as an easy exit from these feelings.

When doing clinical rotation in nursing school, I remember watching a nurse who had to have the narcotics she dispensed checked with another nurse. I was told this was because she had been stealing narcotics for her own use and had been caught. I felt pity for her. Again, I thought to myself, "Not me! Never!"

Eventually, I obtained my RN license and I moved to a bigger town with high expectations of a new career. I started working for a large hospital, and things seemed to be looking brighter. I was making money, and soon I bought a house. I still had no wife or family, so it was easy to fall into a pattern of thinking, well, I might as well drink. And drink.

After working for several years, I found some pills in the cabinet at my parents' house while visiting. They were Vicodin. Ever since learning about these in nursing school, I had had an interest in what it would be like to try them, so I found myself taking one. I really liked the sense of well-being and found them to be what I thought was a direct route to contentedness. I took three bottles of narcotics from my parents, substituting Tylenol for the Vicodin. I was hopeful my parents wouldn't need any pain medication.

When I ran out of my parents' pain medication, I began manipulating the process of distributing the narcotic pills intended for my patients at work. I stole them regularly to make me "feel right" with what I perceived as wrong with my life. I had a couple close calls of being discovered, but that did not alter this behavior. I was not happy unless high. I was stuck with repeated feelings of urgency to self-medicate. Alcohol worked alone if it had to, but eventually I preferred to combine it with narcotics.

As time went on, I changed my position, leaving the orthopedic floor, going to the ER, and managing to go about 6 months without anything but alcohol. Still, I paid attention to how easy it would be to get my hands on the injectables. Then a day came when I did get into those injectables. I had never given myself shots before. I remember it felt natural and exciting to sneak a partially used vial of morphine and try it out. I started out giving myself IM shots of narcotics, preferably Dilaudid. I soon became addicted and eventually began IV use. I would steal the vials, keeping them in my socks, occasionally giving myself a shot at work to help make the night go more smoothly. After a while, I would attempt to procure enough for the time away from work, even working overtime to get more. I realized I was addicted and tried over and over to stop by myself, but was unable. It seemed impossible. It was a dark time for my soul. I had transient thoughts of suicide. I developed a morbid outlook on life and had to get high to cope. This became progressively worse over about a year and a half.

One day, impending catastrophe came my way when I was called to a meeting with the director of the ER and DNS after working a night shift. I was not entirely surprised by this. I was confronted and subsequently fired. I faced a crisis I had never come close to experiencing in my life. I was in denial, and there was such a feeling of panic, as if a dark storm were upon me after my having felt its approach for years.

An individual whom I worked with called me because she had noticed my disappearance from work. She was part of a support group for recovering nurses, and she told me she had had a similar dismissal years prior. She left me a message of hope that started my recovery. I think this is what formulated the prospect that I needed others and could not do this alone.

Initially, I was in intensive group therapy, in which I was active for about 18 months. After completing that, I became a regular member of a support group for recovering nurses, the one my coworker had called me about. At first, I did not particularly want to do this but afterward found it to be very helpful in ways I could not have imagined. Its participants were nurses, and the topics focused on nurse-centered issues. In the process, I made friends, and through this group I was able to embrace my disease like I had not in the other group I had been in. The meetings encouraged participation in a more relaxed way than I was used to. The group members were a lot like me, and I felt as though I was able to use my disease as a strength to help others. I found myself developing insight on how to handle life as a nurse, a loved one, and just a member of society. I don't always handle my feelings well. Working in a program for recovery, letting my feelings out, seeing them for what they are, help me manage them in a healthy way.

I feel that using is not an option for me today, but I know that strength lies in humility—knowing I am fragile. I have also found that helping others is key to my happiness and that the best insurance an addict like me can have is to participate in recovery with others.

Today, I am very thankful that I am able to experience a new way of living and a new way to deal with my problems and to be more accountable to others. Being fired led into recovery and forced me to deal with a nightmare I was unable to escape on my own.

Being accountable to my sponsor and the outpatient group I was involved in became a sort of safety net for me, which allowed me to develop healthy tools and work a program of recovery. The first few months were quite difficult for me, but as time went on, life in recovery got easier. I credit my early success to my choice to not fight. As the Big Book says, acceptance is the answer. The insight, support, and understanding I got from other nurses who had been in recovery longer than I helped greatly. I followed instructions. I read the Big Book. I had a sponsor.

Once I was back to work several months later, I had support, which helped me see how important it was to be accountable to others and myself. Life today as a nurse requires me to be accountable at all times to myself and those with whom I work. Helping others understand the disease of addiction has always been useful. When appropriate, I talk openly to others about what I have been through. I cannot afford to dismiss my past if recovery is to continue into my future.

References

Alcoholic Anonymous. (2013). *The big book* (4th ed.). Retreived from http://www.aa.org/bbonline/.

Alcoholic Anonymous Australia. (2013). Glossary of Terms. Retrieved from http://www.aa.org.au/new-to-aa/glossary-of-terms.php#Unique

American Psychiatric Association. (2000). *Diagnostic and Statistical Manual of Mental Disorders*, 4th Edition. Washington, DC: American Psychiatric Association.

American Society of Addiction Medicine. (1990). *ASAM news*. Retrieved from http://www.asam.org/docs/asam-news-archives/1990-3-4vol5-2ocr.pdf?.2

Baird, C. (2011). Prescription drug abuse: Just the facts. *Journal of Addictions Nursing, 22*(1–2), 72–74. doi:10.3109/10884602.2011.547021.

The Betty Ford Institute Consensus Panel. (2007). What is recovery? A working definition from the Betty Ford Institute. *Journal of Substance Abuse Treatment 33*(3), 221–228.

Ettner, S., Huang, D., Evans, E., Ash, D., Hardy, M., Jourabchi, M., and Hser, Y. (2006). Benefit-cost in the California Treatment Outcome Project: Does substance abuse treatment "pay for itself?" *Health Services Research, 41*(1), 192–209. Retrieved from http://www.ncbi.nlm.nih.gov/pmc/articles/PMC1681530/

Gaufberg, E., Barnes, R., Albanese, M. & Cohen, P. (2009). *A faculty development workshop for primary care preceptors: Helping your residents care for patients requesting opioids for chronic pain.* Cambridge, MA: Harvard Medical School/Cambridge Health Alliance (Massachusetts Consortium).

Goldstein, E. (2012). The neuroscience of bad habits: Dr. Nora Volkow. *The Huffington Post: Addiction and Recovery.* Retrieved from http://www.huffingtonpost.com/elisha-goldstein-phd/bad-habits_b_1501477.html

Grohol, J. M. (2007). 15 common defense mechanisms. *Psych Central.* Retrieved from http://psychcentral.com/lib/2007/15-common-defense-mechanisms/

Hart, P. D. (2004). Faces and voices of recovery public survey. Washington, DC: *Faces and Voices of Recovery.*

Kleinig, J. (2008). Recovery as an ethical ideal. *Substance Use & Misuse, (43),* 1685–1703.

Myers, D. (2002). *Insufficient justification effect.* McGraw Hill Online. Retrieved from http://highered.mcgraw-hill.com/sites/0072413875/student_view0/glossary.html

National Council of State Boards of Nursing. (2011). Appendix H: Definitions. *Substance Use Disorder in Nursing* (pp. 236–239). Chicago, IL: National Council of State Boards of Nursing

National Council of State Boards of Nursing. (2011). Introduction and purpose. *Substance Use Disorder in Nursing* (p. 3). Chicago, IL: National Council of State Boards of Nursing

National Council of State Boards of Nursing, Substance Use Disorder Committee. (2011). *Substance use disorder in nursing. Return to work guidelines.* Retrieved from https://www.ncsbn.org/SUDN_10.pdf

National Institute on Drug Abuse. (2010). Drugs, brains, and behavior: The science of addiction. *NIH Pub* No. 10-5605. Retrieved from http://www.drugabuse.gov/sites/default/files/sciofaddiction.pdf

Rosen, S., Miller, T., and Simon, M. (2008). The cost of alcohol in California. *Alcoholism, Clinical and Experimental Research, 32*(11), 1925–1936. doi:10.1111/j.1530-0277.2008.00777.x

Star, K. (2011). Magnification and minimization: Your cognitive distortions contributing to panic? About.com: Panic Disorder. Retrieved from http://panicdisorder.about.com / od/

Substance Abuse and Mental Health Services Administration. (2011). Results from the 2010 National Survey on Drug Use and Health: Summary of national findings. NS-DUH Series H-41, HHS Publication No. (SMA). 11–4658. Retrieved from http://www. samhsa.gov/data/

Trinkoff, A. M., and Storr, C. L. (1998). Work schedule characteristics and substance use in nurses. *American Journal of Industrial Medicine*, (34), 266–271.

Wickizer, T. M., Krupski, A., Stark, K. D., Mancuso, D., and Campbell, K. (2006). The effect of substance abuse treatment on Medicaid expenditures among general assistance welfare clients in Washington state. *Milbank Quarterly, 84*(3): 555–76. Retrieved from http://www.ncbi.nlm.nih.gov/pubmed/16953810

3

getting back to work

This chapter explores early treatment and reentry into the job market—what to expect if you are attributed with an SUD, what to consider, and how to prepare for returning to work in early recovery. Licensing considerations are discussed, such as the fact that standards vary from state to state, as well as fundamental distinctions between discipline approaches and alternative-to-discipline programs.

Prevalent Perceptions

Even though you know the medical definition of SUD, if you are new to recovery, it can be nearly impossible to avoid the self-judgment and cultural stigma that accompany this disease. After hitting bottom, if you are burning up with embarrassment and fear, you may feel like you've crash landed back on Earth. While you're confronting a mess of emotions, finances, legalities, and prejudices, the DSM V definition may not mean much to you. One of the benefits of the road to recovery is shifting from stigma to understanding and well-being. No matter how much you feel alone and overwhelmed, there is help for you and the millions who are also living with the consequences of this disease.

Substance abuse is an issue of epic proportion costing heartache, lives, and billions of dollars. As noted in Chapter 1, "The Bottom Dropped Out," SUD statistics for nurses correspond to national statistics (NCSBN, 2011, p. 2). This refutes any presumption of professional immunity from the disease of addiction. We are now at a critical threshold. If cultural and professional denial and attitudes of ignorance, avoidance, blaming, and shaming don't shift, it is make-believe to think the costs surrounding addiction will just melt away. More likely, numbers will continue rising over the next few years, as they have in the past. Looking at drugs alone, not including alcohol, overdose death rates in the United States have more than tripled since 1990 and have never been higher. A 2011 report from the Centers for Disease Control (CDC) stated that in 2008, there were 14,800 prescription painkiller deaths (CDC, 2012).

Standing on a ridge between archaic reactions and professional attitudes, nurses need a vital, viable, and educated approach to recovery. Buckle your seatbelt. Countdown commencing. Here is your opportunity to become better educated and more proactive regarding this national health issue by way of your own recovery journey. While gaining traction in recovery, you become a role model and a mentor to others by default. Perhaps that is why you're reading this book: You want to be the change.

Your attitudes and approach can infect others. Your infection will weaken or strengthen the disease model for personal and professional recovery. If you're living with an SUD, your healing path will boost a deficient system. But first things first. Take your own medicine. Ensure that you do what you need to do to recover. Do that, and one day your antibodies will permeate the system.

Granted, the culture is slow to change. Noteworthy proponents of the disease paradigm have existed since 1804, when Thomas Trotter published "An Essay, Medical, Philosophical, and Chemical, on Drunkenness, and Its Effects on the Human Body." He wrote that "the habit of drunkenness was a disease," and moreover, "a disease of the mind." In 1909, Oscar Jennings published "The Re-education of Self-Control in the Treatment of the Morphia Habit," which explained that addicts were not willing victims but sick people whose will lay dormant "because of a psychosomatic affliction" (London, 2005).

With the onset of Alcoholics Anonymous (AA) in the 1930s, the disease model gained more credibility. So nearly two centuries after Trotter's essay, why isn't it more common to find institutional and cultural applications based on the scientific methodology of disease when it comes to addiction? The contradictory meld of perceptions comes from a clash of beliefs. Science says that addictive behavior results from a disease, some religious perspectives consider it a sin, and social propriety deems it a weakness that can lead to unethical or illegal actions.

It is easy to miss diagnosing the symptoms of this disease because they show up as ethical and moral violations, including lying, stealing, and cheating. They can also include breaking the law, breaking hearts, and breaking trust. You already know this if you are suffering from an SUD. You have violated your own moral, and perhaps ethical, code. For most people, that is what it takes to get help. The symptoms are costly—not just for the patient but also for family, friends, and employers. Allowed to go unchecked, the quality of care and patient safety are compromised.

Jean

During my intensive outpatient program (IOP), we had a lesson on core values. The counselor asked, "How many core values did you violate during your disease?" Oh my goodness, was I shocked. I had been stealing and lying. When using, I never looked at myself in the mirror and thought, "Yep, I lie; yep, I steal." I was an addict through and through. I didn't think I needed help, either. I went into rehab kicking and screaming. I was glad when my IOP was over, but I learned a lot—a lot more than I expected.

State Programs: Alternative and Discipline

If you have recently been attributed with an SUD and you want to retain your nursing license, you will fall under the scrutiny of your state's board of nursing (BON). Each state has its own process and set of requirements, which are based on state law. State programs fall into two general categories: One category follows a rehabilitative approach and the other follows a traditional disciplinary approach.

Although almost 90 percent of state nursing boards offer an alternative-to-discipline program, a minority of states still enforce a discipline model. These programs are referred to as *punitive, dismissal, discipline,* or *traditional discipline.* Programs and agency policies that offer an approach based on a disease-treatment model for rehabilitation are designated as *alternative to discipline, alternative to dismissal,* or simply *alternative.*

As noted by the NCBSN SUD manual:

> The Substance Abuse and Mental Health Services Administration
> (SAMHSA) reported that only 14 percent of Americans addicted
> to alcohol and drugs actually seek treatment for their addictions
> (SAMHSA, 2008). But it was not until the 1970s and 1980s that
> addicted nurses were even offered treatment prior to disciplin-
> ary action (Torkelson, Anderson, & McDaniel, 1996). Although
> the condition, substance use disorder, was already considered a
> treatable disease by the American health care system, the disease
> concept was not widely extended to the addicted health care
> provider. Nurses and doctors were denied the same nonpuni-
> tive approach being offered to the patients they served. Many
> of these providers did not receive treatment until after they had
> been criminally charged. This mindset began to change when
> boards of nursing petitioned state legislatures to approve diver-
> sion legislation. The new legislation made it possible to offer
> treatment to addicted nurses without having a negative impact
> on their licenses as long as they continued to meet certain re-
> quirements. Forty-one states, the District of Columbia, and the
> Virgin Islands have since developed programs to channel nurses
> with a substance use disorder into treatment and recovery pro-
> grams, monitor their return to work, and prevent their licenses
> from being revoked or suspended (NCSBN, 2011, p. 2).

With 88% of state boards following an alternative-to-discipline methodology there seems to be nationwide support for the rehabilitative approach
to SUDs. There is growing substantiation that this approach is actually
safer for the public. "The public gets more protection when health-care in-
stitutions offer an alternative-to-dismissal policy. Such a policy can get an
impaired nurse off the job and into treatment within days to a few weeks,
while documenting the proof to terminate employment can take years"
(Monroe & Kenaga, 2011, p. 505).

Regarding alternative approaches, the National Council of State Boards of Nursing (NCSBN) states, "Alternative to discipline programs is a successful alternative to traditional disciplinary approaches. Each state is given the power to regulate professionals such as nurses within their jurisdiction and to let boards of nursing use their professional expertise to enact rules or regulations and to implement and enforce the statutes relative to the practice of nursing in their state" (NCSBN, 2011, p. 38). The NCSBN does not regulate, but rather performs an advisory role for each state's board of nursing. The mission of the NCSBN is to provide education, service, and research through collaborative leadership to promote evidence-based regulatory excellence for patient safety and public protection (NCSBN website, 2013).

Alternative-to-Discipline Programs Versus Disciplinary Approaches

Alternative programs usually:

> Have the nurse refrain from practice. This can be for a designated period while the patient undergoes early treatment and establishes evidence of sobriety and a recovery program.
> Establish a program for monitoring workplace fitness.
> Require random or regular UAs (urinalysis for toxicology screen).
> Require a psychiatric evaluation.
> Have restrictions that are progressively lifted at intervals when sustained abstinence is demonstrated.
> Require support group attendance (for example, AA/peer support).

Disciplinary approaches may be identified by the following:

> They commence due process.
> If the nurse is found guilty after due process, the nurse's license is suspended or revoked.
> No state board recovery program is offered for nurses with SUDs.

Throughout everything, it is critical that the rights of the public and the rights of the nurse be balanced because professional discipline of any type can jeopardize a nurse's career and livelihood (Raper & Hudspeth, 2008). Two key pieces of information you'll need to know are as follows:

> **Does your state have a disciplinary or an alternative-to-disciplinary approach?** You can get this answer from your state's board of nursing (BON).

> **What is your employer's policy?** Your employer's policy regarding substance infractions may or may not be congruent with your state board's approach. Employers more commonly respond with a punitive or automatic-dismissal policy. With considerations of reputation, insurance, safety issues, and staying in business, the impulse for any agency to react swiftly and strongly to violators of ethical and legal standards is currently a reality. For example, at the time of writing, the Idaho Board of Nursing (IBON) follows a Just Culture model. The Just Culture model was articulated by David Marx in the 1990s to describe an institutional attitude that is balanced between a punitive and an enabling approach to employee mistakes.

Regarding substance abuse and addiction, the NCSBN SUD manual (2011) states the following:

A Just Culture environment changes the response to the nurse's addiction while accountability for the addiction is maintained. The fact that the alternative program is not punitive does not mean accountability is ignored. Nurses who enroll in an alternative program are accountable to themselves, their program monitor, their counselors and other nurses, their work-site monitors or supervisors, and are held responsible for abiding by the contract they signed upon entering the program (NCSBN, 2011, p. 51).

In testimony to the United States Congress, Leape said:

> Approaches that focus on punishing individuals instead of
> changing systems provide strong incentives for people to report
> only those errors they cannot hide. Thus, a punitive approach
> shuts off the information that is needed to identify faulty sys-
> tems and create safer ones. In a punitive system, no one learns
> from their mistakes (Leape, 2000).

To further illustrate the importance of knowing both your state's policy
and your employer's, let's look at Idaho, an alternative-to-dismissal state,
as a case in point. Regardless of the Idaho Board of Nursing's (IBON) policy
supporting rehabilitation, two notable hospitals have practices that oppose
each other. One actively supports a therapeutic recovery model for nurses
who committed workplace infractions due to SUDs; sometimes, while demonstrating compliance of contract or upon completion, the nurse remains
eligible for rehire. The other hospital, which describes itself as being unpar-
alleled in nursing, may theoretically support the DSM-V definition of substance use disorder, but in practice opts for automatic dismissal of nurses
who have diverted with no possibility of rehire. Even though this type of
institutional hypocrisy promotes hazardous underreporting of SUD issues,
the point here isn't to hide substance abuse from your employer. Just know
that if your state BON has a recovery culture, your employer might not
share the same philosophy. (Note that this example is through the authors'
direct experiences and interviews with current and former staff nurses associated with the hospitals. This is not intended to be a scholarly comparison;
rather, it is a real-world anecdote of how things sometimes work.)

Employment Variables in Your State

As someone in the early stages of recovery, your ability to retain or obtain
work depends on whether you reside in a state with a disciplinary or alternative policy. Most states have alternative-to-discipline laws. If you are in
or moving to one of the few disciplinary states, you could be automatically
red-flagged for the remainder of your career. This adverse career brand can

follow you from state to state. Furthermore, as Jane discovered in the following story, it is valuable to know if anything that you disclose in any format (letters, emails, cover letter, and so on) can be publicly divulged.

Jane

I was in love and wanted to move to another state and get my license there so I could work! I contacted the state's board of nursing, but they seemed resistant to talking to me. The woman said, "Well, we don't have a program," as if she was trying to deter me. I wasn't getting the clue: "You're going to get denied." And that's what happened. I applied and they denied me licensure.

When I applied, they asked me to write a letter about my history. I wrote a very candid letter about my history from the age of 16 on. I included what I had done for recovery and where I was today. I read it to two people who were important to me in recovery. Both said, "That's very candid, but that's a clear picture. That sounds good. I think you should send it. It gives them an idea what recovery really is: what we talk about in meetings, what happened, what it was like, and how it is now." I sent the letter off to them, and they sent me back a denial letter. That went on my record. The whole thing—the letter and denial went on the Internet!

I had to spend $7,000 on an attorney to dispute that. The state's board of nursing was not willing to give me licensure unless I would be on probation. Apparently, this was very light compared to what they really wanted to require. My attorney said that it was an excellent deal for me to be on 2 years' probation, have random UAs, and be red flagged on the Internet. I was good with the probation. As for the UAs, I was already 3-plus years into a monitoring program. But it was hard to swallow being branded with the Scarlet Letter! To this day, if you go to Nursys to validate my RN license, you will find a red warning symbol next to my name in that state.

CAUTION *In a traditional disciplinary state, speak with an attorney before making any decisions or declarations.*

Generally, people who are addicted don't tend to seek treatment until they hit bottom. However, with workplace interventions, there are nurses coming into treatment before they've hit bottom. Some of these nurses eventually understand how bad their addiction really is and end up embracing recovery. Others front working the program. Obviously, if you want to keep working as a nurse in a traditional disciplinary state, it will serve you to get into recovery before you're discovered on the job. That said, the thrall of addiction usually trumps good sense. Remember that there are options for help, which include the following:

> A confidential employee assistance program (EAP) counselor

> An intensive outpatient program (IOP) for treatment

> A 12-step program like those provided by AA and NA; call the hotline or main office for information (visit http://www.aa.org, http://portaltools.na.org/portaltools/MeetingLoc/, or http://www.na.org/?ID=phoneline to find the number of the chapter in your area)

> A drug/alcohol counselor

> An MD or psychiatrist who specializes in addiction

NOTE | *For further information on these options, read Chapter 4, "Treatment Options."*

Ryan

I remember thinking rehab was going to be overwhelming. I also started to realize, "You don't have very many choices left here. This is your life right here and now. It's either this or you've got nothing." When I started learning some things about myself, I actually enjoyed it. I'll admit, it took a long time. Sometimes I thought it was a pain. But I could never repay the debt for the knowledge that I got about myself through treatment. You can't put a price on that, you just can't. I think that I get more out of AA, but the treatment was still invaluable. The last part of treatment was more a cognitive self-change class. It got repetitious, but they are trying to effect a change in somebody. Change doesn't happen for people like me overnight.

Questions to Ask Regarding SUDs

> What does my state's Nurse Practice Act require?

> What is my employer's policy?

> What are the confidentiality policies for my state regarding my employment?

> Who, if anyone, is required to have knowledge concerning my license/restrictions?

> Where can I find answers? Good places to start include your organization's human resources department and your BON's website.

Treatment and Monitoring Contracts for Licensing

For nurses identified with an SUD, what types of requirements might be included in an alternative program? State board contracts generally include evaluation and monitoring. Some contracts may require that you participate in a treatment plan. Monitoring can be administered by the state BON staff, a BON-contracted agency, a professional association, a peer-assistance program, or a state agency other than the BON, such as the department of health.

While requirements vary from state to state, one thing you can count on is being surprised and, at times, offended. Initially, some of the monitoring requirements may seem outlandish, unnecessary, and expensive. Over time, however, many nurses in recovery have gained an appreciation for these life-saving requirements. If arrested and convicted, be prepared for additional requirements such as meetings with your parole or probation officer, jail time, or alternative programs such as work release and/or drug court. Drug court is "a special court given the responsibility to handle cases involving drug-using offenders through intensive judicial supervision, case management, mandatory substance abuse treatment and drug testing, and graduated sanctions and rewards" (Akron Municipal Court, 2012, p. 4).

It can be overwhelming when you are first facing the requirements and total expense of the state's monitoring program. For instance, if you retain a paycheck but not a driver's license, it can appear overwhelming to get to all the required meetings in 1 week: three treatment appointments, one UA, one peer-support meeting, and two 12-step meetings add up to seven meetings in 1 week. And this does not include additional meetings with a monitor or appointments at drug court! If you've lost your job, then you have time for meetings but may appear to be lacking the finances to pay for them along with living expenses. Either way, it can be stressful—and stress is one of the things that got you here in the first place!

Tom

The nursing board and program for recovering nurses (PRN) created certain restrictions to help protect patients and allow nurses to continue their careers. These limitations are in the contract nurses sign when they join a PRN. Most participants are familiar with them, but the constraints that can easily create trouble are narcotic restrictions and working night shifts or overtime.

Employers and coworkers often do not understand the significance of PRN nurses needing to adhere to these restrictions. They may simply think the nurses are difficult, needy, and not team players. PRN nurses might be asked to pass narcotics, work night shifts, or work overtime, even though their workplace monitor knows they are not yet allowed to do so. In such cases, it is up to that PRN nurse to explain that he or she is not able to perform such actions. The results of going outside of the parameters of your contract can be dire.

NOTE *There is an AA expression: "First you come, then you come to, then you come to believe." It is normal to feel stunned, scared, and overwhelmed. Just know that many before you have made it through and have come out on the other side. A formula for success includes following good counsel and taking the next step. Another AA expression goes, "Do the next indicated thing." That is all you need to do.*

Remember the board of nursing prime directive to keep the public safe? Well, that has a lot to do with alternative program protocols. At times, it might feel like you are being punished by having certain duties stripped away and restrictions installed. The intention is to reassure the public that it is safe while giving you another chance. You get the opportunity to detox your body, heal your brain, institute a recovery lifestyle, learn new tools, and reduce relapse risks.

Most newly recovered civilians stay away from bars and big party scenes, but you may work at the scene of your crime, and an early return to work is like entrapment. You are set up for failure, and your employer is set up for betrayal. This is not a test of willpower. It is a disease with a full set of workplace liabilities. If you have something to prove to yourself or anyone else by getting your job back, you've already failed. You can't prove you have something you don't have. You can't spontaneously develop immunity to the disease of addiction without recovery. So, first understand that the plan is to get you out of harm's way until you understand well enough what you're up against and are better equipped to make healthier choices. Think of it this way: Would you hire someone who is deathly allergic to bee stings to work at your bee farm? Regardless of how much she loved bee farming and how much protective clothing she wore, the answer would be no! In spite of her pleas, you would drive her off your property as fast as possible.

If you are a participant in an alternative program, your journey might go like this:

1. You will be removed from risk, at least in the workplace. This both removes you from harm and keeps patients and coworkers safe. This might involve a transfer, suspension, or dismissal.

2. You undergo psychological/psychiatric evaluation to help determine your fitness and the parameters for the contract.

3. You sign a contract with your state's board of nursing.

4. You establish evidence of abstinence and evidence of adherence to the contract. Evidence includes the following:

    > Compliance with terms of contract

    > Attendance at scheduled UAs

    > Clean UAs (possibly observed)

    > Attendance at required treatment, including inpatient/outpatient treatment program, 12-step meetings, working with a sponsor, and nurse peer support groups

    > Compliance with work restrictions

    > Reports from workplace/site monitor

    > Attitude of willingness versus denial

    > The obtaining of permission and maintenance requirements when traveling

If your license is suspended, you have a break from workplace traps and triggers and time to establish new habits, such as going to support groups, working with a sponsor or counselor, establishing alternatives to substance use, and so on.

5. You apply to your BON or monitor to return to work with a limited license. Typically, there are designated time frames before you can apply to your monitor for a limited-license work return. A limited license has specific workplace restrictions, which preclude handling narcotics; working overtime, nights, or weekends; floating to other units; and working in the ER, critical care, hospice, and home health.

6. You apply to your BON or monitor for the removal of restrictions. Restriction removals are based on cultural wisdom and statistical results regarding time frames, compliance, and your particular history.

7. You maintain evidence of abstinence and compliance for the designated duration of the contract. State board contracts generally vary in length from 1 to 5 years, depending on infractions, duration of abuse, psych evaluation, and the state BON's program. There is evidence that nurses are less likely to relapse after participating in a 5-year program versus a 3-year program. According to the NC-SBN, research supports increased monitoring contracts as a way to increase long-term success. "The findings from one study recommended the length for the contract for monitoring be extended from 3 to 5 years" (NCSBN, 2011, p. 106). With regard to contract duration, be aware that if you relapse, you may be required to restart. This is often determined by your monitor and the severity and number of relapse(s). For example, if you relapse 3 years into your 5-year contract, you can be required to add 5 more years onto the 3 you've already completed. If you suffer multiple relapses and noncompliance with your contract, you may be disqualified from the program.

8. You become part of the solution by assisting others in recovery. This will happen over time. As you gain footing in your new life, you will naturally reach out to help others in peer support groups and 12-step groups such as AA/NA.

NOTE *Costs during this period can include psychological evaluation, out-patient or inpatient treatment, regular UAs, peer-support group dues, monitoring, and being unemployed or underemployed.*

Reconcile yourself to the fact that there will be pleasant and unpleasant surprises. Surprises will come in the form of unanticipated expenses and windfalls, unanticipated breaks, and requirements you never anticipated. Some will come packaged as people who are supportive and others as people who are skeptical and unsupportive. Regardless of the challenges, if you are dedicated to recovery, you will find support when you least expect it and most need it. All the other challenges help reprogram your perceptions and reactions. For more tips to prepare you for the mental and emotional intensity of the recovery journey, see Chapter 5, "Recovery: Getting It and Keeping It."

NOTE *Many tools and groups offer support and guidance to help you succeed in recovery. This doesn't mean everyone you encounter in the legal arena, BON, or workplace will be civil or helpful, but enough individuals and groups want to help you recover. If you have a sincere desire, the help will be there.*

There are many unavoidable frustrations in this journey. To minimize self-induced frustration and misunderstandings, use the cover-your-rear principle. Make an electronic and hard copy folder to track all correspondence with your monitor. When working with a monitor regarding your contract, make sure everything is in writing, including the following:

> Any details that are important to you

> Anything you are told that matters to you

> Any pending change to your contract, including time frames

In addition, for your records, summarize all verbal conversations into email form and send them to your monitor for written confirmation. For example, if on the phone your monitor approves your vacation request and agrees to suspend UA testing for that time period, immediately compose and send an email to your monitor that says something to this effect:

Dear Monitor X,

I am writing to confirm your approval for my travel request to Maui from February 13–20. You have also suspended my requirement to submit a UA during that time period. During this travel period, I have agreed to attend a minimum of five AA meetings and have my card signed. I will submit to a blood test upon my return if so requested. Please write back and confirm or edit this summary. I will book my flight when I receive your written confirmation. After 3 years in the treatment program, I feel ready to travel with my family. We have already located the AA meetings and I have reached out for a temporary sponsor while on the island. His name is Bill, and his phone number is XXX-XXX-XXXX. Let me know if I have left out any other instructions to maintain my contract compliance.

Respectfully,

Y

Changes in Employment Protocols

Early in your recovery, you may remain employed, remain employed with restrictions, be suspended pending investigation, or have employment terminated, with or without the option for future rehire. Regardless of the details, you will experience change. Even if you retain a job with your current employer, there will be adjustments. For example:

> You may experience a shift in your role, position, schedule, or duties, which may result in a decrease in pay.
> You may be required to report to a work-site monitor.

> Your restrictions may be disclosed to your manager and/or coworkers.

> Your coworkers' duties may be affected.

> You may face resentment or distrust from coworkers.

If, in the early stages of your recovery, you find yourself searching for a job, think about a few things:

> **Your résumé.** What is the best format? What are employers looking for in today's competitive market?

> **Interview skills.** What should you say—and what should you avoid—in interviews? When and how much should you disclose? (For guidance, see the next section.)

> **Where should you apply?** Should you stay in the industry or opt for nonindustry employment?

> **What position do you want?** Do you want to work full time or part time? Consider your capabilities and the physical and mental toll of SUDs. What are you mentally and physically capable of right now? It takes the brain and body time to recover from chronic substance abuse.

> **Volunteering.** This may offer opportunities for employment in the future.

> **When should you apply?** Is it better to stay unemployed or underemployed while getting grounded in recovery? There is no right answer when it comes to convalescence and time off.

The guiding principle is to do what best serves your life-support program of recovery. For some, this might mean an extended break from work; for others, it might mean working part time and taking a break from self-preoccupation. Home stressors also factor into the equation. Depending on your circumstances, it may be more taxing to spend too much time at home than to be a part-time barista or shelter volunteer.

TIP *If you are seeking general guidance and employment support, see Chapter 7, "Careers and Change," for a link to a self-guided career-coaching template. This resource includes tools for writing your résumé, interviewing, and sorting out what career direction is best for you.*

Regardless of the particulars, the circumstances that most threaten your recovery are the ones you should mitigate. Substance use disorder is a life-threatening consideration. Remember the character who is morbidly allergic to bee stings? In your case, you can quite literally work yourself or indulge yourself to death. The good news is that you don't have to figure this out on your own. In fact, *don't* figure it out on your own. That would be ill-sought advice. One of our AA friends says, "Every time I have a good idea, I tell my sponsor. And then we figure out how bad it really is." In early recovery, as with being under the influence, impulses are cross-wired. Judgment is suspect and often impaired. Your recovery team will help you sort out what is most supportive for successful recovery. The longer you recover, the better your judgment will become. Eventually, you will be able to trust your motives and your decisions. That can take years.

CAUTION *The more you want to resist counsel, the more key seeking counsel may be to your recovery. Ask yourself, "How long has my judgment been compromised?" The next time your peer support group tells you to pause before applying for your old position, and you find yourself more interested in telling them why you're ready than in listening to their concerns, you can be pretty sure you're under the influence of impaired thinking. With your life on the line, are you too busy having all the answers to listen to people who want to keep you alive? Many new addicts have felt guilty for so long that defensiveness is a common response to anyone who doesn't immediately endorse early recovery plans. Your recovery team didn't show up to make life more difficult for you. If you stop and consider that your recovery team is giving you what they believe is lifesaving advice, you can realize that they aren't trying to thwart your happiness. This isn't Mom and Dad saying you aren't old enough to get your ears pierced.*

SUDs and Recovery Disclosure: Who, When, and How Much to Tell

In early recovery, disclosure can feel like being forced to expose your naked self. It can feel risky. Will you be penalized if you don't disclose? Will you be penalized when you do disclose? There are so many factors that determine your fate. For example, you can never be sure of the personal bias of a manager or interviewer. Trying to guess the outcome of your declaration gets you no closer to the result than to move forward. Unlike hiding your addiction, the road to recovery is paved with honesty and openness.

Just know that reactions to SUD disclosure come in all flavors. They can vary from denial ("Nah, you don't really have that big a problem") to disbelief, judgment, pity, horror, overzealous sympathy, encouragement, and neutrality.

Whether you're wondering about disclosure in your current workplace or in the interview process, it is always advisable to consult an attorney, your state board, and the agency about your rights and requirements. The same questions apply:

> Whom to tell
> When to tell
> How much to tell

If you're facing disclosure in your current workplace, you'll likely need to speak to your manager. In this case, two different scenarios with potentially different outcomes exist:

> **You have a substance abuse issue and are entering recovery.** In this case, advise your employer beforehand that you have some weighty news, and that you would like him or her to take time and consider your information before responding or taking significant action.

> **You have a substance abuse issue, you are entering recovery, and you have committed related workplace violations (worked while impaired, diverted, etc.).** In this case, your employer will most likely have to take immediate action.

If you're deciding if and when you should disclose during an interview, the general rule of thumb is to be up front. That said, don't jump in *too* quickly. Being up front doesn't mean you disclose it in a cover letter. You also need to know what is legally required by your state BON or recovering nurse program. You want to know what your recovery team advises, and you might want to consult an attorney.

TIP | *Chapter 5 covers the steps for disclosure in early recovery. These steps include being prepared, getting guidance, letting things simmer and settle, and being compassionate. Chapter 7 further addresses disclosure and prejudice.*

After a long spell of substance abuse, it is typical to experience mortification. Extreme emotion can prompt rash behavior. You might feel compelled to blurt out inappropriate confessions or move underground—anything to block painful feelings. Pop quiz: What do you do when you can no longer resort to numbing out with a life-threatening substance? If you answered, "Call someone on my recovery team and ask them how to ride out the storm," you got it right!

CAUTION | *Take careful note of extremes in your reactions. Proceed with caution if you feel inclined to tell everyone or to tell no one. (For more on disclosure, self-recrimination, and paying penance, see the section "Disclosure: Who, When, and How Much to Tell" in Chapter 5.)*

Disclosure is all about setting the stage—preparing yourself to to deliver the news about your disorder in the most appropriate fashion and then accepting any response you receive. Then you discover how the next chapter of your life will unfold. It's a mystery worth investigating. Regardless of the outcome or the other person's reaction, if you have followed your recovery program and applied good guidance, you are likely to experience a renewed sense of peace, freedom, and self-respect.

Serenity Prayer

God grant me the serenity to accept the things I cannot change; courage to change the things I can; and wisdom to know the difference.

–Reinhold Niebuhr, adopted for use by AA/NA

Job Readiness

Aside from the logistical issues (when and where you can work), more substantial issues of self-preparedness and recovery fitness exist. Are you physically, mentally, and emotionally fit to work at this job under threat of relapse due to triggers? If you're quick to answer that question, you've probably got the wrong answer. If you pause to think about it, you might come to get it right. For more specific questions to appraise your recovery and job readiness, see the section "Questions to Ask Yourself" in Chapter 7, "Careers and Change."

Rosie

At the beginning of my recovery, the first thing I thought I had to do was get busy. "Let me just get back to normal; let me just get back to work." That was the only thing that I really cared about for probably a good 6 to 9 months. Later in recovery, I realized it's not healthy to go back to work too soon. It would have been disastrous for me to jump back into the same environment.

Recognizing when you're far enough along in your recovery to return to nursing requires clearing out the ego, the autopilot, and the control issues, and overriding the impulse to run back to the disaster zone. This is an journey of maturity, wisdom, and dedication to your long-term best interests.

Maybe you're wondering, "If I can keep my job, should I?" or, "If I can qualify and get hired for that job, should I take it?" If so, in a brilliant, lucid moment, answer this: Will this job be a good fit for your recovery? When are you healthy enough to know what is best for your recovery? That is not a rhetorical question. Measure that answer in years (not days, weeks, or months). Then go ask your recovery team.

No matter how much you tell people that you have recovery handled, in the first few years most motivations for wanting to retain or replace an old position are fear based. How long has it been since your motives have been addiction free—5, 10, 15 years? If you are willing to consider a career change, you're on the right track. It is not that you *have* to change careers; it is more about being willing to put your recovery first and your work second. If you are willing to walk away from your job to save your life, you have the proper priorities and a better chance of "working a good program."

When a person with SUD stops using drugs, it does not mean that his or her thinking process automatically shifts from addictive rationalizing to rational thought. Even if you never abuse drugs again, it can take months or even years to become more reasonable and less reactive. When it comes to career considerations, if you're automatically rationalizing why you should charge back into work, this most likely isn't coming from a healthy perspective. There is a thinking disorder that accompanies addiction that makes it difficult to learn from pain. Take Sally for instance. When Sally rode the roller coaster at age 35, it made her nauseous. Riding roller coasters lost all its appeal and she never was tempted to ride them again. However, when Sally wakes up nauseous and hungover and vows never to use drugs again, a few hours later she turns a 180. By the time she pulls into the parking lot at work, she's already fantasizing about the way she's going to feel when she takes pills she's going to divert during her shift. Rationalizing, blurring reality, and the misguided confidence of addictive thinking says, "Going right back to work is a great idea! In fact it's the best idea ever!" Do you really think that all those workplace triggers will no longer seduce you?

Karen

I had a job interview when I was 10 months into recovery. It was with a new surgeon moving to town, and it was exactly like the position I had lost due to diversion. The interview went well, and I was offered the position. When we discussed my monitoring program, the doctor was very supportive and still willing to hire me. Then he asked me, "How will I know if you're relapsing?" And I could not answer that question!

I was so intent on having that job. I felt like I had to prove to myself and everyone else that I could do that job. I was okay. I could handle it. You'd see. I was still a good nurse. I know now that it would have been a disaster for me if he had offered or if I had accepted that position. I would've been walking back into a hornet's nest. I hadn't yet dealt with any of the issues that had kept me using. I was still horribly codependent and a people pleaser.

Instead, I found a job in medical research. It opened a whole new field I never would have considered. I stayed in that position for 3 years. It afforded me a well-needed break from exposure to narcotics. It also gave me an opportunity to have a schedule conducive to going to AA meetings, having random UAs, and generally getting some tread in recovery.

If you have recently stopped abusing drugs or alcohol, you are one big, exposed nerve. You are no longer numbed by drugs and hangovers. You have higher levels of emotional, mental, and physical sensitivity. What used to be tolerable may become intolerable—especially before you develop healthy coping skills. Workplace circumstances that used to seem routine can now adversely affect you. For example, the death of a baby or a five-patient trauma can stir greater emotional reactions than previously experienced. Why do you think you used in the first place?

Geri's Story

I was reared in a family where drinking was a very natural thing. We didn't go fishing without beer, we didn't know holidays without drinking, drinks at night, all of that stuff. Wine was my drug of choice. I'm grateful that I didn't have the added burden of narcotics addiction. I never got a DUI but should have. I never lost a job, but I came damned close. I didn't lose my relationships, but the potential was certainly there. In some ways, I guess I was a high bottom drunk, but from the inside I wasn't. It isn't how much you drink or what it does to you on the outside; it's what it does to you on the inside. I was drinking and unable to sleep at night until I about passed out. I would get my first drink when I got home, and I would drink until it was time to go to bed. My husband would go to bed. I would stay up. I never drank in the morning, but I drank later and later into the night until it was almost morning.

I was in a management position. In the beginning, I came at 7 in the morning so I could see my night staff. I'd be there in the afternoon when my 3–11 staff came. That way, I got to see all my staff. The impact of drinking on my work was, if I didn't have a meeting early in the morning, I would call and say, "I'll be in a little later." I'd get there by 10 instead of 7. Things got worse. My clinical nurse specialist came to me and said that she'd been chosen by my management staff to talk with me because people had complained of smelling alcohol on my breath. I thought about that, and I just thanked her. I can't believe I did that, but I did. I thanked her for having the courage to talk to me. That night I'd only had two drinks. Only two. Of course, I had good size glasses; that saved me the walk to the fridge!

The next day, my boss knocked on the door, pulled me out, and took me into my office. I was put on suspension pending investigation. He had the employee health nurse outside the door. She took me to draw blood and do a urine test. I was devastated. I was scared, not so much for myself in that moment but for my family, because I was making most of the money. When I got home, I called back in and talked with the employee health nurse. I knew I had a problem. It had been something that had been worrying me. So there's a piece of me that surrendered right there. But I still was negotiating.

She got me an appointment to see a counselor and talked to me about the nurse monitoring program. This was a Friday. It was really tough being suspended on a Friday and feeling hung out over the weekend. I hope other nurses are given information so they know whom to call and what to do next. I was nearly hysterical by the time my husband got home and I told him. Truthfully, he was relieved—scared, but relieved. He'd been worried, but he's a great enabler. I made him sit down and said, "I don't know what's going to happen or what I'm going to do, because I could lose my job with this." It turned out that I signed a piece of paper for the hospital that said if I ever drank again, I would be fired. So all of that is part of my surrender piece. I had to have an evaluation, and the recommendation was outpatient treatment. I didn't realize how sick I was, so I did the outpatient.

It was helpful that management was so kind. That whole business of suspension pending investigation allowed me to save a little bit of face. I felt that they dealt with my staff very well. Only the people who had to know, knew. I'm sure people may have suspected. They knew I was sick; they knew it was serious. They didn't know when I was going to come back.

In my treatment program, I realized that no matter the position held at work, the person is sick. You are not well. That was a good concept for me to grasp. There is something about my makeup that does not allow me to metabolize alcohol the way that other people do. Part of that makeup is chemical, and part of it is mental. Thinking over my life, I always felt like I was on the outside looking in. I never felt a "part of" things. Now, when I'm in a meeting, I'm a "part of" things. I understand people and situations here, and people understand me in a way that my husband doesn't. I've made peace with the fact that he never will. That's okay. Now when I need an AA meeting, I get a stack of dollars on the table from him. That says, "You get your butt to a meeting!" He doesn't say anything, it's just… he understands that's a part that makes me better.

One of the hardest things for me in treatment was when we did family stuff and I sat knee to knee with my daughter. She recounted drunken episodes and how unsafe she felt driving in a car with me. This is my child. She remembers being unsafe. She remembers so much that I didn't think she did. That was one of the hardest pills for me to swallow. So many of us selfish drunks go to that place where we don't think we're hurting anybody but ourselves.

I realize now I was really protected, and that was an important gift! I think that it's important that people have that kind of protection. I had the benefit of my sick time and got paid the same as if I were working. I mean, what a gift. I am grateful that I was able to keep my job and my marriage.

References

Akron Municipal Court. (2012). Drug court: A program offered through Akron Municipal Court and Oriana House, Inc. Retrieved from http://courts.ci.akron.oh.us/programs/drug_court.htm

Centers for Disease Control. (2012). Policy impact: Prescription painkiller overdoses. Injury prevention and control. Retrieved from http://www.cdc.gov/homeandrecreational safety/rxbrief/

The Grapevine. (1950). The Serenity Prayer. *The International Journal of Alcoholics Anonymous.*

Just Culture. (2000). Testimony of L.L. Leape, United States Congress.

London, M. (2005). History of addiction: A UK perspective. *The American Journal on Addictions, 14*(2), 97–105.

Monroe, T. and Kenaga, H. (2011). Don't ask don't tell: Substance abuse and addiction among nurses. *Journal of Clinical Nursing, 20*(3–4), 504–509. doi: 10.1111/j.1365-2702.2010.03518.x

National Council of State Boards of Nursing, Substance Use Disorder Committee (2011). Substance use disorder in nursing. Return to work guidelines. Retrieved from https://www.ncsbn.org/SUDN_10.pdf

Raper, J., and Hudspeth, R. (2008). Why board of nursing disciplinary actions do not always yield the expected results. *Nursing Administration Quarterly, 32*(4), 338–345.

4

treatment options

You are going to need help. Either you decide this, or someone will decide for you. What type of help will you get? Some choices will be optional, and some kinds of help are mandatory. You may not like any of them, or you may want to get an A+ in all of them. Indeed, typical responses to recovery and treatment cover a wide range:

> I don't need any help. There's nothing wrong with me or my life.
> I'm willing to do anything. I can't keep living like this.
> I'm hopeless and helpless. There's no way I can get out of this mess or stop using.
> I can do this on my own.

This chapter tells you how and where to get help, including resources and types of treatment available. This chapter clarifies some standard recovery nomenclature. It also touches on recovery plans: what they mean and the importance of using them.

Choosing Recovery

Some of you have committed fully to recovery. Others may continue in denial. Denial can sound like, "Maybe I have a *wee* bit of an issue, but I don't need to be put in the same category with those losers in AA." "Or, my offense wasn't *that* bad. Those three DUIs could have happened to anyone. There were 5 years between each one. Who *doesn't* overindulge from time to time?" Or, "What I do on my own time doesn't have anything to do with my job." You may be right, but is it worth your quality of life and professional status if you're wrong? You don't have to decide anything now. Just keep reading and listening and staying curious.

If you are ambivalent about nursing and recovery, you are not the first. Many before you doubted their need for recovery but half-heartedly decided to give it a try. That decision can be a lifesaver—or at the very least, a career saver. After all, if you fail to recover, you will mostly likely have to surrender your nursing license.

Most nurses decide to continue on a path to recovery. What happens next? Each state has the capability to impose regulations and restrictions. These are covered in each state's Nurse Practice Act. These rules define the scope of practice for nurses and assist the nurse in determining what is considered misconduct, unprofessional conduct, incompetence, or being unfit to practice (National Council of State Boards of Nursing, 2011, p. 25). If you are entering the recovery path or questioning whether this is the road you want to take, you will need to have some information about treatments and programs available.

Standard recovery options include the following:

> Employee assistance programs (EAPs)
> Support groups, such as 12-step programs (Alcoholics Anonymous [AA] and Narcotics Anonymous [NA]) and peer support groups
> Inpatient treatment programs
> Outpatient treatment programs
> Individual counseling

When you're sincere about recovery, you will find life providing you with support. Think about the brazen determination and perverse perseverance that came naturally to you while using. Nothing could stand between you and your endgame. When you were under the spell of addiction, not using simply wasn't an option. The options were, "When do I use?", "How much can I use?", and "Where do I use?" When you weren't using, you were plotting. Now think about putting half of that determination into recovery. If you want recovery, then not recovering is not an option.

These primary strategies support success:

> Recognize that you can't stop on your own.
> Seek appropriate guidance. This guidance comes from those who have gone before you and have successfully lived in remission from SUDs (a.k.a., recovered from addiction). Your guides will become your recovery team. With help, you never have to use again.
> Take action. Carry out instructions.

> Be persistent. Follow AA's advice: "Do the next indicated thing." Remember this, also: "It's progress, not perfection" and AA's counsel to "Keep coming back" (Alcoholics Anonymous, 2001).

To review, you can do this:

> Chuck it all and leave nursing.
> White-knuckle it and try to do recovery on your own.
> Follow the state board of nursing (BON) mandates to retain/regain your license and enter a treatment program.

If you opt for the last option—and we hope you do—be aware that mandatory requirements are generally stated in a contract with your monitoring agency. (For some examples, refer to Chapter 3, "Getting Back to Work," in the section "Treatment and Monitoring Contracts for Licensing.") Options are limited, and include the following:

> Which approved treatment center you enroll in. You may or may not have a choice of attending an inpatient or outpatient program. Inpatient programs are more like intensive care, while outpatient programs are more like regular dialysis treatments. Generally, if you want a controlled environment for early sobriety, opt for inpatient treatment. If you are deemed at higher risk—say, you have suffered multiple relapses—you may be required to attend an inpatient program.
> Where you attend 12-step meetings.
> Whom you select for a 12-step sponsor.
> Which nurse peer support group you attend. These are support groups distinct from 12-step programs, intended for nursing professionals who share specialized occupational challenges to recovery. Of the approved groups, you decide which one to attend.
> Additional individual counsel. This includes work with a therapist (psychologist or psychiatrist) or a recovery coach. If you have an EAP, you often have access to a counselor.

Employee Assistance Programs (EAPs)

EAPs are an employee benefit offered by many larger companies. They provide one-on-one support as well as initial assessment and intervention for problems at work or home, including those related to substance abuse. EAPs allow a limited number of visits and will make referrals to community resources, such as individual counseling or intensive treatment programs. A team of nurses at the Indiana University School of Nursing (Godfrey, Harmon, Roberts, Spurgeon, McNelis et al, 2010) found that "hospitals with employee assistance programs were relatively more likely to facilitate the reintegration of recovering nursing employees. In order to optimize success, a recovering nurse needs to be surrounded by a supportive work environment" (p. 2).

NOTE | *EAPs are not full treatment programs. They are listed here because an EAP can be a good starting point for help and direction.*

Support Groups

Support groups are the foundation of recovery. While the result of participating in support groups may feel therapeutic, they are different from therapy groups in that they are not usually facilitated by a therapist or a drug/alcohol counselor. They are most often facilitated by peers who have long-term sobriety and who have the ability to impart reliable recovery practices. Therapy groups are the mainstay of intensive in/outpatient treatment programs. Individual counseling, discussed later in this chapter, is an optional adjunct to support groups and intensive treatment.

Support groups include 12-step programs and peer support groups. Often, attendance at support groups is required to augment inpatient and outpatient treatment. Because addiction is considered a disease of isolation, support groups offer a number of social and recovery benefits. In groups, people help themselves by helping others. Participants also feel accountable to the group, which can help them maintain sobriety.

When people are active in their addiction (abusing drugs or alcohol), more and more of life happens in the shadows. Many addicts become undercover agents, hiding behaviors and desires from others, all the while becoming more disconnected, irritable, irrational, defensive, untruthful, and moody than healthy people. When a drug becomes your one true companion, you might have become unreliable and inconsistent at showing up to social and family functions. People don't call as often. When you were using, were you more self-preoccupied and less aware of the needs of others? Part of the payoff of relinquishing the substance is connecting with others and belonging to a community. The feelings of support, being valued and understood, and contributing can help fill the unrelenting void of abstinence.

12-Step Programs

A 12-step program is considered a key component of most treatment programs. The most common are Alcoholics Anonymous (AA) and Narcotics Anonymous (NA). In particular, AA is recognized worldwide as the premier recovery program, and attendance is free. According to the AA website, it has 114,070 groups worldwide with over 2 million members. The United States has 58,820 groups with over 1 million members. Many state BON contracts require or suggest that you attend AA or NA to supplement treatment. In these 12-step programs, success is determined by participating in the program and experiencing a reprieve from the compulsion to drink or use. A key premise is that by helping others to stay sober, you help yourself. In AA's own words:

> Alcoholics Anonymous is a fellowship of men and women who share their experience, strength, and hope with each other that they may solve their common problem and help others to recover from alcoholism. The only requirement for membership is a desire to stop drinking. There are no dues or fees for AA membership; we are self-supporting through our own contributions.

AA is not allied with any sect, denomination, politics, organization or institution; does not wish to engage in any controversy, neither endorses nor opposes any causes. Our primary purpose is to stay sober and help other alcoholics to achieve sobriety (1980, p.3).

NA puts it this way:

The group atmosphere provides help from peers and offers an on-going support network for addicts who wish to pursue and maintain a drug-free lifestyle. Our name, Narcotics Anonymous, is not meant to imply a focus on any particular drug; NA's approach makes no distinction between drugs, including alcohol. Membership is free, and we have no affiliation with any organizations outside of NA including governments, religions, law enforcement groups, or medical and psychiatric associations. Through all of our service efforts and our cooperation with others seeking to help addicts, we strive to reach a day when every addict in the world has an opportunity to experience our message of recovery in his or her own language and culture (2012, ¶ 1).

There are two main types of AA and NA meeting designations:

> **Closed meetings.** These are most common. As defined by AA, closed meetings are only for those who have a desire to stop drinking or using.
> **Open meetings.** Anyone is welcome at an open AA or NA meeting. If you are hesitant or just curious, go to an open AA or NA meeting. There are no requirements to attend. To find a meeting, call the AA Intergroup or visit http://www.aa.org. For NA, visit http://portaltools.na.org/portaltools/MeetingLoc/.

If you are uneasy or fearful about going to your first AA or NA meeting, you are not alone. Most people don't *want* to go to that first meeting. If you haven't been to a 12-step meeting, here is what you can expect:

> Meetings generally occur in churches or businesses but are not affiliated with any business, sect, or denomination.

> Many meeting rooms are accessed through an alley or side street instead of through a main lobby. If you're unsure which door to use, ask someone heading toward the building if they know where "friends of Bill W." are meeting. Bill W. was one of the founders of AA. (This is handy when you are traveling—for example, on a cruise or at a resort. You will see a note in the activities log or on the meeting-room door: "Friends of Bill W. meet here.") When looking for NA meeting rooms you can ask for "friends of Jimmy K." This stands for James Kinnon, who founded NA in 1953.

> You'll see many different types of people and a range of demographics: students, homeless people, executives, grandparents, and so on, and they will be dressed up or down and out. All are united in a common purpose: the desire to stop.

> A chairperson opens meetings. At a designated time, the meeting chair will ask, "Are there any newcomers? If so, please share your first name." This isn't to expose or embarrass you. It allows other members to make your acquaintance, answer questions, and connect you to other helpful members at the end of the meeting. Everyone in that room can remember his or her first meeting.

> Meetings generally follow a topic identified by the chairperson. You can share about the topic or on anything else that will help you stay sober. You do not *have* to talk or share, however. If asked, you can state that you would rather just listen.

> You are strongly encouraged to find a temporary sponsor who can introduce you to the program and the culture. You've made a good start when you begin to recognize the similarities between your story and those of others. The old ego/addict thinking focuses on the differences between you and everyone else. AA calls that *terminal uniqueness.*

> If you don't jet out the instant the meeting ends, people will intro-
duce themselves or offer their phone numbers. Generally, women get
numbers from women and men from men. (You can ask your temporary sponsor why this is the norm.) Armed with phone numbers, the
hotline, and a meeting list, you have ready help if you're tempted to
drink or use.

TIP
*For more information, read AA's online pamphlet, "A Newcomer Asks"
(http://www.aa.org/pdf/products/p-24_anewcomerask.pdf).*

Al-Anon

Al-Anon and Alateen are not for recovery from substance abuse. Rather,
they are support groups for people who have relationships with people with
substance abuse issues. Al-Anon and Alateen are recovery programs for the
spouse, friends, and relatives of alcoholics (codependents).

Al-Anon members say that those who love a practicing alcoholic become
as sick as the drinker. The main purpose of participation in Al-Anon is not to
help sober up the friend, lover, parent, child, or spouse, but to free the codependent from his or her own destructive behaviors. Although it shares
some of the same principles of recovery as AA, Al-Anon is a separate
entity and is not affiliated with AA. While not necessarily a goal of Al-Anon,
those in the program feel that if they become healthier and change how
they behave, they can help the alcoholic to a new awareness (Missouri
Department of Social Services, 2006). It is not uncommon to find recovering
addicts or alcoholics who are parents, friends, and spouses of other addicts
or alcoholics attending Al-Anon.

Aubrey

You might run into a lot of misconceptions about 12-step meetings from your family and friends. I took my husband to an open AA meeting because he didn't know what went on there. He thought we stood up with sunglasses and told fake names and stuff. I invited him to come to a meeting with me. So we kind of made it a date night. Afterward, as we were driving home, we were talking about it. He realized it wasn't some funky cult where I had to drink the Kool-Aid.

Having been around for more than 7 decades, 12-step programs are successful support group options and universally considered solid recovery choices. In addition to the AA and NA programs, there are fledgling models, such as SMART Recovery; faith-based programs, such as Celebrate Recovery; and Internet-based programs, such as Women in Sobriety. You should confirm in writing with your monitoring agency that any support group you consider attending meets the requirements of your BON contract.

CAUTION

While attending your support groups and deciding which inpatient or outpatient treatment program to enroll in, be advised that just because a provider qualifies for the approved state BON list, it does not mean it offers high-quality treatment. In every professional area, there is a range of acceptable performance. Think of doctors: Experience and expertise vary. The same goes for treatment groups and counselors. If you want the best treatment, do your research. Ask for recommendations from people in your support groups. A common description of a higher-quality program is, "They're tough but they're good!"

If you're not really sold on recovery, you might base your enrollment on logistical factors such as shorter treatment duration, fewer sessions required, or lower cost. You might be affronted by the thought of attending 3 nights a week for 3 hours each *and* as many 12-step meetings, plus homework. "That's just crazy!" you think. "Who has time for that?" The answer: *You* do—if you want to shift away from a life filled with secrecy, shame, and numbness. As noted by the National Institute on Drug Abuse:

> Good outcomes from TC [therapeutic community] treatment are strongly related to treatment duration, which likely reflects benefits derived from the underlying treatment process. Still, treatment duration is a convenient, robust predictor of good outcomes. Individuals who complete at least 90 days of treatment in a TC have significantly better outcomes on average than those who stay for shorter periods (2002, ¶ 2).

Peer Support Groups

According to White (2010, p. 2), "Peer-based recovery support is the process of giving and receiving non-professional, non-clinical assistance to achieve long-term recovery from severe alcohol and/or other drug-related problems." Boisvert, Martin, Grosek, and Clarie (2008, p. 205) concur: "Evidence suggests that a peer-supported community program focused on self-determination can have a significant positive impact on recovery from substance addictions."

The *peers* referred to here are nurse and nursing-related professionals. In any recovery support group, people gather to share experience, strength, and hope. Nurse peer support groups provide an avenue to further address distinct work-specific traps, triggers, and recovery strategies. Some specific traps and triggers include the following:

> Working around the old "candy dispenser" (a.k.a. Pyxis)
> Hearing someone shake a pill bottle
> Smelling alcohol wipes
> Snapping an ampule
> Dealing with arrogant, imperious, or unhelpful colleagues

Working in environments riddled with opportunity and constant reminders makes peer support particularly significant for nurses. According to SAMHSA:

> Peers encourage and engage other peers and provide each other with a vital sense of belonging, supportive relationships, valued roles, and community. Through helping others and giving back to the community, one helps one's self. Peer-operated supports and services provide important resources to assist people along their journeys of recovery and wellness (2012, p. 6).

Peer support groups are most often led by a designated facilitator or coach. As noted by the Substance Abuse and Mental Health Services Administration (SAMSHA):

> Peer recovery support coaching is a set of non-clinical, peer based activities that engage, educate and support an individual successfully to make life changes necessary to recover from disabling mental illness and/or substance use disorder conditions. The activities that comprise this service are education and coaching. A key element contributing to the value of this service is that peer recovery support coaches appropriately highlight their personal experience of lived experience of recovery (SAMHSA, 2011, p. 1).

Intensive Treatment Programs

The two main types of intensive treatment programs are inpatient and outpatient. They are considered intensive in that a concentrated time is spent focusing on recovery practices and confronting issues that promoted abuse and could trigger relapse. This can bring up a lot of uncomfortable and even painful feelings. The core method of this intensive treatment program is centered on therapy groups facilitated by drug/alcohol counselors.

Some programs may employ additional trained specialists who assist with adjunct issues such as anger management, abuse, PTSD, nutrition, exercise, and meditation. A common therapeutic approach used is cognitive-behavioral therapy.

Cognitive-Behavioral Therapy (CBT)

Cognitive-behavioral therapy (CBT) is based on the cognitive model of emotional response. According to the National Association of Cognitive-Behavioral Therapists, "Cognitive-behavioral therapy is based on the idea that our thoughts cause our feelings and behaviors, not external things, like people, situations, and events. The benefit of this fact is that we can change the way we think to feel/act better even if the situation does not change" (2010, ¶ 4).

Inpatient Treatment Programs

With inpatient, or *residential* treatment, you live at the treatment facility for a specified duration, immersed in the recovery community. Both group and individual sessions are offered.

The advantage of an inpatient treatment program is that it removes you from easy substance access. You can also disengage from the stressors at home or work to focus solely on your recovery. Classes help you develop coping strategies and build new habits. In addition, these facilities often offer other holistic modalities such as meditation or animal therapy.

Treatment stays vary from a 3- to 12-day detox, up to a 90-day therapeutic program. An industry standard is 28 days. (Remember the Sandra Bullock movie by the same name?) Inpatient therapy is more likely to be recommended or required for people with any combination of the following:

> Long-term addictions
> Multiple substance abuse

> Numerous relapses
> Dual diagnosis
> Repeated legal offenses
> Needing medical detox

Outpatient Treatment Programs

Intensive outpatient programs (IOPs) have the same goal as inpatient programs: to help a person achieve sobriety and freedom from alcohol/drug abuse. The average IOP spans 12 weeks and includes 9 to 12 hours per week in required sessions. Occasionally, you might find full-day intensive classes offered. Major topics include relapse prevention and the biology and psychology behind addiction. With the frequency of abuse issues and post-traumatic stress disorder (PTSD) in people with addictions, some facilities offer separate male and female groups. Individual counseling and family counseling can also be incorporated. IOPs allow you to integrate treatment into day-to-day living.

Martin

I liked my IOP. I was ready for a change. I realized long before I entered IOP that my decisions weren't benefiting me. I had had two DUIs. I knew I had a problem, so I did not go reluctantly. I was looking forward to it, and I had a good time. When you get into a group and there are people working toward recovery and looking at themselves honestly, it's pretty cool. I'd walk out of class and think, "This is a really cool subculture that I didn't even know existed." You can't tell anybody not in recovery your story. Nobody else gives a damn. But you can share with those people in rehab. The ability to share common ground and experiences has been important to my recovery. Like they say in the Big Book, there are certain people who are constitutionally incapable of being honest with themselves—and if you can't be honest with yourself, then you're going to have a horrible time in IOP.

Elizabeth

When I got to IOP, it was a bit of an eye opener. I knew I had to do the program. Not just go through the motions, but really do it. I was old enough to be the mother of most of the kids in my group. And it was such a mixed bag of people, all culturally different. There were meth heads, potheads, and alcoholics. Getting to know those people was a unique experience. I became attached to my group quickly. Even those young kids were amazingly insightful and interesting to watch.

I did my genealogical tree and looked at all the addiction in my family. We had to write down a family timeline. I was shocked when I saw how much abuse and addiction there was in my family, on both sides. It was amazing. I thought, "Damn, I'm lucky I wasn't in here 25 years ago." I learned a lot. From day one I understood I had a disease and had made some bad choices that got me into my seat in treatment. I was so scared when I first walked in, I was shaking. But still I followed instruction, did the next indicated thing, and showed up at treatment.

Individual Counseling

If you are under contract for treatment with your state BON, most likely individual counseling is not a singular treatment option. Primarily, it is not considered as effective in treating addiction as group therapy. One important reason is that group therapy serves as an antidote to the addict's tendency to isolate, and isolating is a major characteristic of addiction. The deeper you go into your disease, the more detached from society you tend to become. Fear of being discovered, along with antisocial tendencies, promote seclusion. In one-on-one counseling, you remain singular and special in your process. In group settings, you acquire peers, and you learn to do the following:

> To realize that you are not alone nor special in your issues

> To socialize

> To support others
> To share a bond with others

When it comes to substance abuse, the therapeutic community favors group therapy. One advantage of group therapy is the cost; it is generally much less expensive than one-on-one counseling. Less obvious are the encouragement and accountability that come with group therapy. As noted by the Substance Abuse and Mental Health Services Administration (SAMHSA):

> The natural propensity of human beings to congregate makes group therapy a powerful therapeutic tool for treating substance abuse, one that is as helpful as individual therapy, and sometimes more successful. One reason for this efficacy is that groups intrinsically have many rewarding benefits—such as reducing isolation and enabling members to witness the recovery of others—and these qualities draw clients into a culture of recovery. Another reason groups work so well is that they are suitable especially for treating problems that commonly accompany substance abuse, such as depression, isolation, and shame (2005, p. 1).

In an interview, one counselor said, "Everyone benefits from listening to the person in the 'hot seat.' In addition, one-on-one therapy is so expensive!" That being said, the counselor went on: "If, 2 or 3 years from now, the addict still has incest or abuse issues or PTSD, and she can't get through it with a sponsor in her fourth or fifth step, or hasn't seen a psychiatrist for meds, then that's a different story. She probably does need additional counseling."

If there is unremitting trauma, individual counseling can effectively augment your treatment plan. One of the major benefits of supplementing group therapy with individual counseling is taking an intensive look at issues that contributed to the need to escape through substance abuse. Many addicts have been through abuse or other trauma and can find more in-depth, one-on-one therapy supportive to addressing preexisting issues.

Unresolved issues are considered a major contributor to relapse by many drug/alcohol counselors and 12-step sponsors. Many nurses develop serious health problems and may suffer from posttraumatic stress disorder, anxiety, depression, or insomnia (Felblinger, 2008). This anxiety and depression may then cause a nurse to turn to alcohol or drugs to deal with the stress (National Council of State Boards of Nursing, 2011).

Two emerging additions to the list of psychology, psychiatry, and counseling include the therapeutic application of EMDR (short for eye movement desensitization and reprocessing) and the use of life coaches specializing in recovery.

EMDR

EMDR is an eight-phase process of resolving past traumas through the use of bilateral stimulation. More than 20 controlled studies of EMDR have been conducted showing its effectiveness in treating trauma and other disturbing life events (Shapiro, 2012).

According to EMDR practitioner Dr. Patricia Morgan (personal communication, May 20, 2013):

> Many times in my practice as a clinical psychologist, I have seen that addiction is more than just an out-of-control behavior, and is affected by other factors, including negative beliefs and negative emotions, and especially the effects of trauma. EMDR is powerful for resolving trauma. An example from my clinical experience: One woman was drinking heavily daily to help her deal with the emotional distress of childhood sexual abuse. In resolving the trauma of that abuse through EMDR, her drive to drink subsided.

Treatment centers throughout the United States and abroad have witnessed the value of incorporating EMDR as an adjunct to their addiction programs.

Recovery Coaching

Recovery coaching offers support and guidance for people who desire recovery from addiction. This includes coaching sessions to reinforce decisions and behaviors that support recovery as well as selecting further treatments such as detox, intensive inpatient/outpatient programs, family support, education, and support groups. Recovery Coaches International describes recovery coaching as follows:

> Recovery coaching is an ongoing professional relationship that helps folks who are in or who are considering recovery from addiction to produce extraordinary results in their lives, careers, businesses, or organizations—while advancing their recovery from addiction. Recovery coaches affirm that there is innate health and wellness in each of our clients. We hold our clients as creative and resourceful. We do not promote or endorse any single or particular way of achieving or maintaining sobriety, abstinence, or serenity or of reducing suffering from addiction. Our focus is on coaching our clients to create and sustain great and meaningful lives (2011, ¶ 1-2).

How to Choose

When it comes to choosing your recovery resources here are some worthwhile considerations:

> If you live in an area with limited resources and you want to broaden your support system, research online groups to supplement. For example, if there's one 12-step meeting with five regular attendees where

you live, and you would like more variety and input, you can find links, discussion forums, telephone meetings, real-time chats, and more on AA's website (http://www.e-aa.org/links/index.php).

⟩ Fortunately, 12-step programs don't charge for attendance and peer support groups usually cost only a nominal fee. That means you can shop around for ones that best support your recovery. Questions to consider include whether the group is solution/recovery focused in its topics and guidance and whether there are attendees in the group who have experienced long-term recovery (measured in years versus days or months). This usually indicates a quality recovery community.

⟩ Are the therapists, counselors, coaches, and/or peer support facilitators experienced with recovery tools and principles? Are they appropriately challenging rather than sympathetic and coddling? (Some of the questions in the next bulleted list apply when choosing an individual counselor.)

There are more factors to consider with regard to intensive inpatient/outpatient treatment due to the greater time, financial expense, and group commitment involved.

Upon intervention, you may be required by the state BON to go immediately to an inpatient facility. When selecting the facility it is important to know the treatment center's philosophy. Ask them questions:

⟩ Do you believe addiction is a disease or a choice?

⟩ What kinds of addictions do you treat or specialize in?

⟩ Is yours a lock-down facility (no visitors allowed)?

⟩ What types of treatment do you offer? Do you offer 12-step programs? Group or family therapy?

Sometimes, the monitoring agency may restrict which facility you can use, so make sure you ask these more practical questions before you sign a commitment:

> Do you provide aftercare (ongoing therapy/support group for those who have completed the intensive treatment)? Is it included in the cost? How much and for how long?

> Are you medically based (have detox capabilities, etc.)? Generally, medical detox will involve an evaluation, including what drugs you're on, in what quantities, and any other diagnoses you may have. Detox attends only to the physical dependency, not the underlying psychological problems that might be present.

> Are you accredited/credentialed?

> Do you offer financing options?

TIP | *If a peer support group is available to you, go! Ask other nurses where they went and what they experienced.*

Most people entering recovery are concerned with finances: How will you pay for all of this? Here, it is important to reframe the question: How can you possibly *not* pay for getting your life back, keeping your career, and saving yourself?

First make an honest assessment of where you are financially:

> Am I still employed? Will my employer assist me?

> Do I still have insurance? Will it cover any (or all) of my treatment?

> Do I have savings or retirement to tap into? (What better way to spend money than on your future health and happiness?)

> Can I get a personal or medical loan?

> Do I have family or friends who might lend me money? (Make it official. Sign an agreement of loan terms. Have them pay the money directly to the facility.)
> Do I have things I can sell?

Now is the time to call in favors. Also, don't be afraid to ask facilities if they can help you. Make sure you get the costs up front and in writing. Just remember, you are not alone! Many have gone down this path before you. Ask how they managed. What did they do?

More About Insurance

With the implementation of the Affordable Care Act in 2014, there may be changes to insurance coverage. At this time, the insurance exchanges are required to include mental health coverage in benefits. In addition, plans should comply with the "parity" law, requiring the same level of coverage as for medical/surgical treatment. (This applies to large employers.) If you can't get treatment through your health insurance plan, consider the following (HBO Addiction, 2013):

> Don't let the stigma of addiction prevent you from fighting for insurance coverage for drug and alcohol problems.
> Most states have laws requiring insurance plans to cover addiction treatment.
> Prepare by becoming thoroughly familiar with your employee benefits and by being ready to challenge any efforts to deny coverage.

Amy's Story

It was about 8 years ago, after my baby died, that I got bad migraines. My addiction started before that, though—I just hadn't recognized it. My doctor prescribed Relpax, but the pills made me feel like I couldn't breathe. That's when I was put on Norco. I remember getting a migraine and, after taking Norco, thinking, "Wow, I feel really good. I could feel like this all the time." It numbed everything. I could do everything without getting headaches. I would take one right before bed. It didn't make me go to sleep, but I remember the feeling it gave me: I wanted to talk to my husband about the whole day. I did that for a few months. I realized that my doctor would just refill them. At the end of the month, I could call it in and he would refill them without having to see me.

I got pregnant again and rarely touched one. Now and then I would take them for my migraines. During this time, I started nursing school. I didn't want to get drug tested, even though I had a valid prescription and I could've gotten away with it. I worked at a nursing home and hospice. I had morphine on me all the time but didn't touch it.

After I got laid off from hospice, I started having arthritis pain. Within 2 weeks, I was almost totally disabled. I had to lean against the wall to get down the stairs in the morning. That's when I went to the doctor. I went to the quick ER. They took my blood; my numbers were crazy. I had rheumatoid arthritis. I made an appointment with the rheumatologist but could not see him for 2 months. I had no medicine. I didn't even have Norco at that time. I went to the ER at 3 in the morning because I couldn't stand the pain! They put me on Norco, and it was really good.

I didn't abuse the first bottle of Norco. By the second month, though, I'd started abusing it. I figured it was okay. I was probably taking six or eight a day. I was only supposed to take four a day. And I lived like that for a long time. Then I got my job at the hospital and started working a lot of hours. I realized how easy it was to start diverting. I started seeing a different doctor that I worked with. He said, "That's not enough pain meds. Who's being so stingy?" and he upped my Norco from 90 to 120. In the end, it was 180 a month.

I was going through all of those meds. I would take two in the morning. Then I could get meds from work, so I could save my own to avoid withdrawals. I would use when I could at work.

I never deprived a patient of meds, but I remember the first time I diverted. A patient was prescribed Norco. I popped them out, went to give them, and she didn't want them. I put them in my pocket and noted she had taken them. We had a little tackle box. I would go through the packets and see what hadn't been given lately. I would sign it out with my name or occasionally another nurse's name.

In the beginning, I didn't do it every day because I was so scared. Then, when I found out how easy it was, it just became routine. I was doing it every day—every single day. There were a couple times I got really brazen. In the bubble packs of the pills, there was an Oxycontin. I'd never taken that, but I knew it was strong. Nobody had taken it. So I just took the whole card, and nobody ever questioned it. Nobody. And I was like, "Oh my gosh! This is too easy!"

I lived like that for almost a year. I thought I was being a good parent because I could do everything. I could work 12, 16 hours, I could go to my kids' schools to help. I didn't really do that much, though, because I was always at work. I would rather work than be at home. And I would stop in at work to say hi. "Does anybody want a day off?" Who does that!? Who wants to work extra shifts?

The last couple of months, after church, I'd tell my husband, "Oh, let's stop by the hospital. I'm going to grab something out of my locker." I didn't think he knew; he never said anything. I was really dumb, actually. I always had sharps with me or syringes. I always left them around so he wouldn't think anything different.

One day I was scheduled to work ED. I was there with another nurse. She wasn't one who just read the numbers and left. If something was used, she knew. The nurse coming on that night was also one of those nurses, so I knew I couldn't take a lot because those two would catch it. We ended up getting busy, but I got greedy. New boxes of morphine and Dilaudid arrived, and each of them had four tubexes taped on top. I started out taking one here, one there. Working the shift, I took four. There were two brand new boxes left. Any other nurse wouldn't have known. When the count came, I kept saying, "I'll count. You can just go home." But she would not go home. I was thinking, "Please, just go home!" I said, "I've had the narc keys all day. Why don't you just let me and S. count?" And she said, "All right, go ahead." I thought she would go in the other room, but she didn't. She sat right there.

She had to have been suspicious. I don't know why else she would've sat right there. S. said, "Wow, you guys used a lot of morphine today." My heart started racing. She said, "No, I don't think I gave any." I said, "Well, maybe one or two." Then they noticed the next box, too, and said, "Oh my gosh all these meds are gone." I knew right then I'd been caught. I was so nervous I couldn't even finish my count.

The nurses went directly to the DNS. The DNS came in and said, "I'm going to do a UA test on everybody." I thought, "Oh my God, what am I going to do?" Then the DNS called HR and they said, "No, you can't test everybody. You have to go through proper channels." I thought, "Oh good, maybe I got away with it." I went home, but of course I didn't sleep very well.

Oh my gosh, it was awful. I just waited. Monday, I took my son on a field trip with his school, and it was awful because I was having withdrawals. I had body aches and headaches and diarrhea. When I got home from the field trip, my daughter announced, "Mom, the police are here." Oh my God. My kids were scared. "What are the police doing here?" I left them inside and went outside. It was a police officer I knew very well. He said, "I was just wondering if you can come down and talk." I asked, "Do I have to stay in jail?" He said, "No, you get to come home." "You promise?" Because I knew right then I was busted. I explained to my kids that I was going down to the police station.

The day after I got caught, I woke up thinking it was a dream. It was so surreal. Then the reality hit me. When my husband got home, I was in bed because I was really sick with withdrawals. He said, "Well, if you'd quit taking all that stuff in your makeup bag...." I asked, "Why didn't you tell me you knew? We could've fixed this before!" I tried to push the blame on him. He told me, "I was scared and I was sad."

I was so frightened. I knew I had to come clean and get clean. I wasn't sure if I could do it with my RA. I didn't know how I could manage. As the months went by, though, it became clear that I hadn't managed anything except my addiction. It was my only focus.

Now, I realize, as scary as recovery once seemed, it has become my lifeline. Recovery has given me clarity, self-worth, focus, and a new beginning. I continue to struggle with my chronic diagnosis of RA. Now I also have a chronic disease of addiction. As with the RA, though, if I take my medicine, my symptoms stay under control. I work closely with my doctor, and I am honest. That is something I hadn't been in a long time.

My nursing support group has turned out to be my most important meeting. I love AA, but the support group is comforting because I'm surrounded by nurses. We are all so supportive of each other; there is no judgment. I get inspiration from seeing the elders in the group: where they started, where they are headed, or where they are now in their lives. It gives me hope. My tears are gone.

References

Alcoholics Anonymous World Services, Inc. (1980). A newcomer asks. Retrieved from Alcoholics Anonymous. (2001). Alcoholics Anonymous, 4th Edition. New York: A.A. World Services.

Alcoholics Anonymous World Services, Inc. (2012, January). Estimates of A.A. Groups and Members. Retrieved from http://www.aa.org/en_pdfs/smf-53_en.pdf

Boisvert, R.A., Martin, L.M., Grosek, M., and Clarie, A.J. (2008). Effectiveness of a peer-support community in addiction recovery: participation as intervention. *Occup. Ther. Int.*, *15*, 205–220. doi: 10.1002/oti.257

Godfrey, G., Harmon, T., Roberts, A, Spurgeon, H, McNelis, A. M., Horton-Deutsch, S. & O'Haver Day, P. (2010). Substance use among nurses. Indiana Nurses Bulletin. Retrived from http://indiananurses.org/isnapsite/documents/2010Godfreyetalfinalcopyf orBulletin_1_.pdf.

HBO Addiction. (2013). Can't get treatment through your health insurance plan? Retrieved from http://www.hbo.com/addiction/treatment/362_not_covered_by_insurance.html

Missouri Department of Social Services. (2006). Substance abuse—Recovery resources. *Child Welfare Manual*. Retrieved from http://www.dss.mo.gov/cd/info/cwmanual/section7/ch1_33/sec7ch16.htm

Narcotics Anonymous. (2012). *Public Relations Handbook.* Retrieved from http://www.na.org

National Council of State Boards of Nursing, Substance Use Disorder Committee. (2011). Substance use disorder in nursing. Retrieved from https://www.ncsbn.org/SUDN_10.pdf

National Institute on Drug Abuse. (2002). Therapeutic community. Retrieved from http://www.drugabuse.gov/publications/research-reports/therapeutic-community

National Institute on Drug Abuse. (2002). The science of drug abuse and addiction. Retrieved from http://www.drugabuse.gov/publications/research-reports/therapeutic-community/what-typical-length-treatment-in-therapeutic-community

Recovery Coaches International. (2011). What is recovery coaching? Retrieved from http://www.recoverycoaching.org/?page_id=11

Substance Abuse and Mental Health Services Administration (U.S.). (2005). Center for Substance Abuse Treatment. Substance Abuse Treatment: Group Therapy. *Treatment Improvement Protocol (TIP) Series,* No. 41. Rockville, MD. Retrieved from http://www.ncbi.nlm.nih.gov/books/NBK64220

Substance Abuse and Mental Health Administration. (2011). Recovery support services: Peer recovery support coaching. Retrieved from http://www.samhsa.gov/grants/block-grant/Peer_Recovery_Support_Coaching_Definition_05-12-2011.pdf

Substance Abuse and Mental Health Services Administration. (2012). SAMHSA's Working Definition of Recovery Updated. Retrieved from http://blog.samhsa.gov/2012/03/23/defintion-of-recovery-updated/

White, W. (2009). Executive summary. Peer-based addiction recovery support: History, theory, practice, and scientific evaluation. Counselor, 10(5), 54-59.

5

recovery: getting it and keeping it

If you're feeling stunned, scared, and overwhelmed, you're on target. To gain a new way of life, you have to dismantle the old one. This chapter emphasizes that recovery is a lifestyle, not a destination. It introduces some useful concepts, tips, and strategies to help you shift into the recovery lifestyle. It also notes some classic pitfalls that you will encounter.

Recovery Is a Lifestyle

Recovery is a journey. And as with any new journey, it is normal to feel disoriented and out of control—something that many addicts just aren't comfortable with. Being uncomfortable has to do with trust issues. The only thing you thought you could really trust is that you would find a way to use or drink. Addicts blow their own ethical moral codes. To be out of control is very challenging when you don't have much faith or trust in how things are going to turn out. A huge part of recovery is discovering how benevolent life becomes when you choose health and well-being.

Many people before you have made it through the discomfort zone and now love their lives of recovery and their recovery communities. As you learned in Chapter 3, "Getting Back to Work," a formula for success includes sticking close to your recovery community, following good counsel, and following this AA maxim: "Do the next indicated thing." Many individuals and groups want to help you recover. If you have a sincere desire, support is there for you. People will say, "It's not always what I want to hear, but it's always what I need to hear."

You can count on discomfort. This pain will not kill you. It will save you. Try to find someone who says that the pain of facing and nullifying her fears did not alter her life for the good. Like a patient undergoing intensive physical therapy, there is a lot of mental anguish and physical pain between the injury and the recovery. Regardless of the intensity and fear of mental, emotional, and physical withdrawal, it is temporary, and there is help to ride the wave. Keep hiding behind drugs and alcohol to avoid pain, and your quality of life will fade. Move through the pain. You will gain a new lease on life and discover or rediscover a person you love being.

These tips can prepare you for the mental and emotional part of the journey:

> **Get qualified support.** This may come in the form of recovery friends, a sponsor, a counselor, a support group, reading materials, and a higher power (as defined by AA). *Qualified* refers to those who model and adhere to proven recovery principles and tools.

⟩ **Follow qualified guidance and the actions suggested.** They work.

⟩ **Expect the unexpected.** When you are abusing substances, it is usual to fear the unknown. While in recovery, you no longer have to cover your tracks and try to control outcomes to avoid consequences. Taking healthy guided action can lead to unanticipated support and benevolence. In 12-step meetings, it is common to hear members express gratitude and give accounts of "miracles."

⟩ **Get comfortable with being uncomfortable.** You are moving into a new way of life. There will be times of disorientation and discomfort. This is good. It will pass if you ride the wave. The pain and fear will dissipate, and you will be liberated into a new life. This is pain with a purpose.

⟩ **Do the opposite of what you're used to doing.** Change old, comfortable—and destructive—behaviors.

With respect to the last point, do the following:

⟩ **Come out of hiding.** With guidance from your recovery team, you will learn how to tell people who need to know about your journey. (You will learn more about disclosure considerations later in this chapter. Some were also covered in Chapter 3.)

⟩ **Reduce isolation.** If you are feeling overwhelmed, vulnerable, or shaky, call someone on your recovery team. This isn't an issue of being strong enough or too weak to get through pain and cravings. It's about learning to reconnect and promote your well-being.

⟩ **Tell the truth.** It has become normal to spin or lie about the truth. Practice telling the truth. This is part of learning healthy boundaries and preventing relapse. Your recovery team will help you learn better communication tools. Authenticity and boundaries are very empowering. You're as sick as your secrets. With trusted allies, you will find grace, healing, and solutions.

❯ **"Practice progress, not perfection."** This AA tenet expresses the idea that consistent and incremental change is the path. Learning to accept your humanity and disease is a huge gift of recovery.

❯ **"Do the next indicated thing."** This AA tenet acknowledges that you can't get it all right, right now. When coming out of denial and seeing a life in ruins, it is typical to want to fix it all—immediately. When you have vision of how things should be and how they really are, you want to start at the finish line. Back up, start at the starting line, and take the next indicated step. You know that recovery and healing are processes. It is the same for reclaiming your life. It takes time. With persistence, the prognosis is excellent.

❯ **Acknowledge the good.** Recovery is about allowing the pain that heals. You also get to recognize the positive changes that occur. When you are overwhelmed, fearful, or uncomfortable, it is easy to blur out all the positive shifts you are making. It is important for your emotional and mental well-being to recognize how you are striding or even inching in a beneficial direction. One way to do this is to reflect on what is different now from when you were drinking or using. An African proverb reminds us, "The rain begins with a drop."

❯ **Call BS on your ego.** Ego is the voice of addiction. It is full of fear and bravado. Its job is to maintain the status quo, even if it is killing you. Ego says, "Change is scary and threatening. Don't change anything. Better the devil you know than the devil you don't." When it comes to recovery, this rationale is terminal. Evidence that ego is present includes the following:

  ❯ Unwillingness or reluctance to change or do something differently

  ❯ Resistance to stepping out of your comfort zone

  ❯ Thinking you are superior to others

  ❯ Believing it is unnecessary to listen to or follow guidance from others ("Because I know more. I'm not that bad....")

  ❯ Thinking you are inferior to others and undeserving

> Thinking you are special and that no one gets you

> In recovery groups, focusing on the differences versus the similarities between you and others

CAUTION *If you are enthusiastic about your recovery, beware grandiose impulses. One trait of addiction is catapulting from one crisis to the next. You've become adept at devising bold strategies to avoid detection and delay the brutal consequences of a life stuffed with chaos and drama. Handling crises and averting disaster can power a hero complex. Combine this bravado with the exuberance of a new (recovery) convert, and the result is a mixture of zeal and a heroic impulse to save the world. First things first: Recover yourself. Then, once you have months and years of traction, you cannot help but mentor change. In other words, slow down. Take things one day at a time.*

Denial: The Emperor Has No Clothes

Elisabeth Kübler-Ross's famous five stages of grief—denial, anger, bargaining, depression, and acceptance—certainly relate to the journey of recovery. Indeed, denial is the overlord of addiction. Harboring denial is like making a deal with the devil. Somehow, you think you're pulling off the impossible while being blind to the astronomical price tag.

Now add your professional culture into the addiction mix. You are a special population with special knowledge, including life-saving education, uncommon coded language, pharmacological knowledge, self-diagnosis, and experience dealing with trauma. In addition, you view drug therapy and ingesting pills as normal, you have a take-charge attitude, you're an authority figure, you exhibit professional detachment, and you're comfortable with needles. Why wouldn't you think you're immune to common diseases? Who hasn't seen a movie where invincible doctors and nurses tirelessly treat patients who are succumbing in droves to contagious diseases? It's enough to shore up any ego.

Denial comes in different forms. One form is that you have outsmarted addiction; therefore, you can bargain for partial surrender. "Yes, I have a problem with opiates, but drinking was never an issue." This is when you hold out that you are not a person with an addictive disposition. You believe that you can specialize and that you are exempt from cross-addiction. It's a theory that many have tried. Another form of denial is a blend of justification and hubris. You've discovered reasons that make it okay to work while you are impaired:

> "I've been doing this for years."
> "I can do this job blindfolded and with one hand tied behind my back."
> "The patients are out of it/comatose/sleeping."
> "It makes me feel more alert."
> "When I alleviate my pain, I am better at dealing with patients' pain."

The addict's convoluted priority becomes not getting caught, never mind patient safety and employee integrity.

Riding the Wave

Without drugs to temper your emotions, they can feel like a tsunami; inevitably those feelings crest and subside. When you get on the other side of the storm, you realize more and more that you won't die. They're just feelings. They're not even reality. They can feel real, but they aren't anything but emotion. Undoubtedly, there have been times in your life when you felt such rage that you said, "I could've killed him!" Did you follow through and commit murder? Of course not. You did something to ride the wave of that amygdala rush to reach calm and reinstate the executive brain function (frontal cortex). Remember: If it was possible *then* to withstand the surge of compelling emotion, it's possible to do so again.

Some might consider this a matter of willpower. Willpower will keep you sick and stuck, fighting for your life. Although willpower looks like it works, it is merely a temporary device to hold back the tide. As a long-term strategy, willpower is no match for the force of addiction. Remember the story about the kid with his finger in the hole in the dyke, holding back the flood? The water pressure never subsides, and the boy is stuck. For life. If he moves, the force of nature will come crashing in. It may begin as a trickle but soon becomes a tidal wave. It's not a matter of *if* the tide will crash into you; it's a matter of *when*. If you're using sheer willpower to abstain from abusing substances, it is not recovery; it's a version of trying to outmaneuver your addiction by controlling it. All clichés apply. It is a wolf in sheep's clothing; the calm before the storm; the dyke before it explodes.

In 12-step programs, there is the term *dry drunk*. A dry drunk is someone who abstains from using and still elicits the mental, emotional, and behavioral traits of someone active in his or her SUD. These include the following:

> Mood swings
> Irritability
> Sensitivity
> Negativity
> Egocentricity
> Victimhood
> Martyrdom
> Intolerance
> Rashness
> Reactionary behavior
> Oppositional behavior
> Justifying behavior
> Dishonesty
> Denial

The good news about living this miserably is that at least you won't be arrested for white-knuckling your abstinence—for making yourself and others miserable. You get to spend your life complaining, and others get to (try to) avoid getting creamed by your self-absorption and negativity.

Employing good recovery tools will give you options, progress, and eventually freedom from compulsion. So what do you do when you feel like you might get sucked back into the gravitational force of planet Zombie Drug User? Put up a barrier to diminish the gravitational pull, and break away. A small action can disrupt the opposing force. It's David-against-Goliath time. Do the opposite of what you feel like doing or the opposite of what you used to do. There was a time you would do anything to indulge your addiction. Now is the time to step further into recovery. Part of recovery is discovering and using your particular spell busters. You have many to choose from. You'll find just a few in the following "instead-of-using (IOU)" list:

> Call somebody. Contact your sponsor, someone in your group, or a supportive friend. Write out their phone numbers on your own IOU list.

> Do your recovery homework. Don't just show up at required meetings; also complete the reading, writing, and step work assigned by your counselor and sponsor.

> Do a thorough first step with a sponsor.

> Apply AA's motto: HOW, short for honest, open-minded, and willing. This reflects the mental state required to change from an egocentric mindset to a mindset open to growth and recovery. Ask yourself a variation of questions based on these principles—for example, where am I not being honest? How am I not open-minded to see an advanced/better/greater/more developed/more mature viewpoint? Where have I been stubborn and unwilling to change?

> Remember H.A.L.T., AA's cautionary acronym to be vigilant when feeling any of the following: hungry, angry, lonely, or tired. The wisdom warns that any combination of those states of being creates more vulnerability to relapse and indicates that it is time to take care of yourself.

> Speak up. Bring up your problem in your support groups.

> Launch a prayer.

> Engage in mindful breathing.

> Journal. Have one handy.

> Write a gratitude list.

> Listen to, read, or watch something inspirational.

> Go help someone. Be of service at your 12-step group.

> Rescript. Change your words and break the spell. "I have a choice...."

Add to the list any additional items that support your recovery:

_____

_____

_____

_____

The list of antidotes to using is long. Your recovery team will introduce you to more tools and resources. The recovery process relies on actions to boost well-being and prevent relapse. Create your own IOU list of actions. Post your list where you can see it throughout the day—on your refrigerator, night stand, closet door, car console, wherever.

Laura

I was worried when we moved out of our house that I would find a pill. I told my boyfriend about my worries. It was kind of funny because when I told him, he said, "Well, if you find something, think of it as poison—or like it's a monster—and that we don't want anything to do with that." Then I went to a support group, and I told everybody what I was thinking. The gentleman running the outpatient support group told me, "If you find anything, let's just make a plan. You're going to get in the vehicle and you're going to drive away from the house—not just go outside but drive away." And I thought that was huge. That really just relaxed me, having a plan. In the end, I didn't find anything.

Restoration

When it feels like the bottom has dropped out, it is particularly easy to focus on how much has been lost, how nothing seems to be working, and how much of a failure you feel. But look again. Have you lost everything? What *haven't* you lost? Better said, what do you have left to lose? Make a list. Go for it. See if you can list 20 things you haven't lost. Here are some examples from others new to recovery:

> Friend(s) who support(s) your recovery
> Spouse/partner
> Child(ren)
> Church group
> Roof over your head
> Good eyesight
> Use of your limbs and digits
> Resiliency
> Clothes
> Enough to eat

> Hope for the future
> Support for recovery
> Employability (if not now, then later when you get deeper into recovery)
> Pet
> Warmth
> The gift of time and recovery
> A sponsor who is there for you
> A peer support group
> Free help (AA, NA)
> Diminished obsession to use
> Hope
> Someone to help you with rides
> A bike
> Hikes
> Time to grieve
> An education
> Cab fare
> Milk money

If you feel overwhelmed and lost now or in the future, list-making is an important tool to shift focus from what isn't working into a field of positivity and possibility. This kind of list is often called a *gratitude list*. Many sponsors and coaches assign a daily gratitude list. At first, it might feel awkward or insincere. If you keep it up, however, you—like many before you—will most likely reap unanticipated benefits.

If you want to shift gears and feel better and more optimistic about your life, you don't have to wait to get an assignment from your sponsor to write a gratitude list. This is a practice you can take up today on your own behalf.

Some people record their lists in a gratitude journal. The list can be 5, 10, 20 items long, or more or fewer. Writing a gratitude list can help you:

> **Repattern from negative to positive thinking modes.** More good comes to those who see the good.

> **Build on what's working in your life.** Life is a self-fulfilling prophecy.

> **Become more spontaneously positive and grateful.** The more goodness you see, the more goodness you get. The more goodness you get, the more you appreciate, and the more support you are able to receive.

> **Recognize that all is not lost.** You have something on which to build.

> **Shift away from self-defeating self-absorption.** Recognize and appreciate how much support, kindness, wisdom, and guidance is available to you.

> **Shift away from being a martyr/victim/helpless/hopeless/ lost cause.** Become a capable human who is able to make positive shifts.

> **Emphasize momentum over inertia.** Recognize that there are positive changes in your life and that you aren't in the same place you were when you were abusing substances. It is easy to miss the significance of these changes when simultaneously facing a mountain of cleanup (rebuilding health, finances, and relationships; maintaining the requirements of your contract; job hunting; etc.). Remember, you don't face it alone. You have your recovery team, support groups, rebounding health, and spiritual resources.

Do not base a gratitude list on grandiosity or hierarchy, qualifying the items for your list based on what might be considered significant or insignificant. The egoic and addictive mentality is fraught with markers of superiority and inferiority. When it comes to developing our ability to experience gratitude and appreciation, all items are valuable. You might be grateful for new windshield wipers, a good cup of coffee, a kind smile, and a coveted job interview. The more you dig for the small gifts, the more you will see what works in your life. The more you see what works, the more you have to build on. These may be small, but they are steps to a greater viewpoint. The climb may be uncomfortable, but the view is breathtaking. One more thing: Although there is no universally correct number of items for your list, try to stop, think, and excavate. This is an exercise that connects you to your good and opens you to greater awareness. It is a marker of recovery and well-being to shift from a limited-negative perspective to a greater-positive viewpoint.

Appreciation and gratitude open you to awareness and receptivity. You first have to be aware to recognize support and gifts. The more you see and receive, the more you can accept that you live in a magnanimous, supportive world.

Jeff

At night, I give thanks for what I've got, and I reflect on the things that happened throughout the day. In the mornings, I ask for what I need.

Rosie

Here's what you do: Anytime you have an opportunity to be grateful about something, stop what you're doing and experience it right then. And then you've got this whole day of gratitude. I've done gratitude lists in the past. I don't need them anymore because my day is filled with experiences that I'm grateful for, and I allow myself to have that gratitude right then.

Disclosure: Who, When, and How Much to Tell

In early recovery, disclosure is a murky zone. Take heart. If you pay attention to people who are years into recovery, they don't seem to struggle with the disclosure topic. Consider it? Yes. Lose sleep over it? No. The longer you stay sober, the more skillfully you will navigate sensitive areas.

People react differently to SUD disclosure. You don't usually get extreme responses, such as people who are overjoyed or overwrought. Instead, people are usually somewhere in the middle: disbelieving, relieved, sympathetic.

Sometimes, you will get the opposite of what you anticipated: A friend who you think will be supportive becomes resentful at losing a party buddy. A boss you think will throw you out of the building offers you encouragement. A mentor turns away. There is no way to predict how people will respond. Although you should communicate in a considerate and constructive manner, you must remember that people are also reacting with their own history of experiences and perceptions. Your part is to set the stage in the most appropriate way possible and then accept the outcome.

Laura

All my friends were crazy drunks. The social outings I went on were all related to drinking, playing darts, playing cards. I went on a cruise all over the world with three of my girlfriends, and the focus of the trip was all centered on, "Where are we going to get our next drink?"

When I told them about going into rehab, they never really sat down to listen. All they were hearing was, "I'm not going to be drinking anymore." I don't hear from them much. I did get a drunk text this week from one of them, "Why are you avoiding me?"

I think we put a face to something that they're afraid of. My best friend for the last 17 years lives and works out of town. She called 2 weeks ago and said, "Are you done with that whole rehab thing? I thought we could go have a drink." I told her I never was going to be done with recovery and I was headed to an AA meeting. But that hurt. A 17-year "friendship," a 17-year using buddy. That was important for me to distinguish. Now I know that these were drinking buddies and not true friends.

Keep this in mind when you are disclosing in early recovery:

> **Be prepared.** This isn't about undergoing hours of research and worry. It's about setting a thoughtful stage without blurting out a desperate confession.

> **Get guidance.** With your recovery team, sort out what and how much is appropriate to say in a given context.

> **Let it simmer and settle.** A first reaction isn't always a true response. Your news might challenge the other person. These exchanges go best when you don't try to control the other person's reaction. Consider how it feels when someone tells you some big news and then tries to control your emotional reaction. Inevitably, there's a reaction to a reaction. Emotion intensifies. Now, consider how it feels in the same situation when you react, blow off steam, settle down, and then can think about it from a higher perspective. When you share, give people time to come to terms with your news. Most likely, it took you years to come to terms with it. Give them a few days to process.

> **Expect a backlash.** You've shared your news, and your friend has responded with smiling assurances that all will be well. A week later, when you call to get together, you get a cool response. What happened? There are so many possibilities. Maybe she realized that she lost a party friend and that you might judge her or expect her to change. Or perhaps she started thinking about all the things she put up with over the years and how much your addiction has cost her. Now that you're showing up present and more coherent, she's safe to let it all hang out. You may have done things that you don't

remember doing. There will be time to address all this. That is why support groups and 12-step programs provide a strong process for cleaning up the wreckage of the past.

> **Be compassionate.** Have compassion for yourself and for the people receiving your news. If you're hurt and scared, they might feel hurt and scared, too.

NOTE

Often, we're so hurt, it is incomprehensible to invite more hurt. During this early period, when you're beating yourself up, it's hard to deal with the possibility of anyone else joining in. This makes it easy to feel fearful of sharing your condition. Get guidance from your recovery team, and then do your best.

If you are mentally (and spiritually) prepared, open-minded, and accepting of the response you receive, then things will usually go better than the worst-case scenario. You might not get the response you want...or you might! It could even go better than you hoped. Whatever the case, it's a character builder. You gain back credibility and face life on life's terms instead of your own drug-induced version. This is a major boost in early recovery.

Disclosure is all about thoughtfully discussing your substance abuse with others. You need to choose an appropriate time and place to explain what has happened in your past and what is going to happen in your future. Then you will discover how the next chapter of your life will unfold. It's a mystery novel worth writing and reading. Usually, if you've done your research and followed good guidance, the conversation will go better than you expect.

VOICES

Recovery is a journey, not a magic wand. When first in recovery, it is easy to feel raw and damaged, and therefore like the injured party. Be compassionate with yourself and those around you. How many years were you navigating life from an impaired operating system? You're not the only one recovering from the effects of your substance abuse—so is your tribe. Give yourself and others the gift of time. Time will reveal the truth of your current choices, whether they be healing or hiding.

Take careful note of extremes. Proceed with caution if you feel inclined to tell everyone or to tell no one. If you feel like a reborn human who can barely suppress the urge to shout your newfound recovery and confess all to the world, slow down. Express your exuberance in your support groups. It is fantastic to have a new lease on life, but it is also unwise to expose newborn skin to everything all at once. In some instances, that exposure can pile on more issues later and open you up to a backlash of emotions. It is wise to minimize emotional upheaval, especially when you haven't yet developed healthy coping skills and can't automatically escape into the old opiate oblivion. Open up and tell the truth when it supports your recovery. Telling the truth requires discernment and guidance. Depending on the audience and circumstance, the truth can require full disclosure or an edited version.

Jo

At dinner, my 12-year-old nephew noticed that I wasn't drinking wine with the other adults. I explained that at one time, I drank too much and developed an allergy to alcohol. So now my body reacts badly to alcohol, and it isn't healthy for me to drink. I went on to tell my nephew if he ever sees his friends drunk, he will be able to notice how their judgment gets impaired. "The more you drink, the more your decision-making shifts from your executive brain to your limbic brain," I said, pointing to the respective regions on both our heads. My dad got interested at this point and replied, "I didn't know that." We went on into an interesting talk about how that shows up as primal reactionary behavior. "It looks like the wobbly guy slurring, 'Give me the keys. I can drive!' right before he pukes on his shoes," I said.

It was time for my nephew to know that his aunt is an alcoholic. But it wasn't time to use the label that carries a lot of connotations and little information. It was more important that he become educated first. We can add the label later, when he knows more about how to use it appropriately. At dinner that night, my family learned more about the disease and how to talk about it in a different way. My nephew didn't have to figure out just yet if it was relevant to tell friends that one of his aunts is an alcoholic. I'm someone he loves who gets very sick if I drink. If he puts it together with the label before we talk about it again, then great. So be it. But at least he started with an educated version instead of a stereotype. And better yet, he has a different take on keggers.

Secrecy, Fear, Shame, and Penance

The opposite of overzealous confession is a vow of secrecy. An excessive need to keep your condition confidential reeks of shame, misinformation, or fear of a prejudiced, punitive world, where you will be verbally or financially persecuted by others if they know of your condition.

Forms of prejudice and repercussions fall on a continuum between mindless and fanatical. Ironically, extreme prejudice is most likely less threatening on a day-to-day basis than the mindless variety. Fanatical prejudice is intentional and deliberate. There are examples of it all over the world toward everything. Does that render you paralyzed and fearful of showing up in the world because someone, somewhere is going to have a problem with something about you? If so, you are living life as a hostage. Extreme prejudice is an exception and occurs in places or cultures that aren't a match for you—not if you want to live a healthy, thriving life where growth and freedom are valued.

Mindless prejudice is more insidious and challenging because it is ignorant and unintentional, and therefore harder to identify and address. The good news is the mindset of one who exhibits this can be shifted with information, education, and patience. Think of your own prejudices and what it would take to open your mind. You can react to prejudice with righteous indignation or understanding. A reaction is an exchange of blows—one jab for another. A compassionate response sounds like, "I don't resent you for your attitude toward me. In fact, it wasn't too long ago that I felt the same way about people with this disease. I am recovering from a life-threatening disease. And while in recovery, I am rebuilding my credibility. Hopefully, in time, you will see that I'm an asset here."

Suppose you wronged a coworker. This could easily have happened while you were unaware and under the influence. Countering righteous indignation with indignation yields more _____ (you can fill in the blank). Often, anger toward others who appear judgmental is a projection of one's own mortification. Human beings would rather focus on how wrong others are than face how wrong they feel about themselves. As you become healthier, you will help build bridges between ignorance and restoration—that is, if you put your recovery first.

Another motive for secrecy is self-loathing. You can't understand that addiction is a disease if you plan to hide your sins from the world until you have righted the wrongs and paid penance for them. Fortunately, you don't have to understand that this is a disease to begin recovery. While this level of mortification is almost incomprehensible, it has a temporary use: It can be the excruciating pain that brings you to your knees. This is the spiritual and psychic surrender that leads to treatment. Feelings of self-loathing and recrimination can be strong motivators to get help. Treatment helps addicts come to terms with this self-loathing and to move beyond it. Without help, however, most addicts opt for relapse.

Although you may intellectually understand that addiction is a disease, you might fear appearing too cavalier to dismiss unethical and immoral behaviors as a result of your disorder. As a result, you may feel the urge to do penance. But regardless of whether people on the outside looking in know it, there is no get-out-of-jail-free card in recovery. When you dedicate yourself to recovery, you embark on a lifelong journey of diligence to your health and liberating service to others. Nothing is dismissed. It is all addressed in due time. With treatment and time, you will come to accept addiction as a disease, not a sin or moral failing. It is a marker of your growth. Recovery means accepting the disease while remembering the cost of relapse.

Annie

If I would say anything to someone in early recovery, it would be to open up sooner and try to get everything out of it that you can. I had to relapse before I "got it." I was always hiding something underneath. I always thought I'd get my A without coming clean. I said what I thought people wanted to hear, and I acted the way I thought I was supposed to act. I wasn't constitutionally honest about anything—not until I went to [inpatient recovery] and they basically beat it out of me. (Well, that's what it felt like.) That's when being honest sunk in.

VOICES

We have to accept this is a disease and monitor it. Compare the disease to diabetes. "Oh, wait a second. It is kind of stupid of me not to monitor this. If my kid goes out Halloween night and is diabetic, am I going to be checking his blood sugar when he comes home? Well, yes. It's just a smart thing to do, and it doesn't mean that I hate him or I think, 'Damn pancreas!'" We have to do this. It goes back to the whole process: Accept it, be responsible for it, and live with it instead of die of it. Motivation and their recovery are states, not traits. They fluctuate, they go up, and they go down. So we shouldn't beat people up or get into a whole lot of blaming, simply because we have to do something different to support them because a state they have has changed.

–Mark H. Broadhead, MD

Rosie's Story

I took two pain pills every day for 9 years. It started with endometriosis. Nobody would give me a hysterectomy or do exploratory surgery, because I was young. They kept saying, "You're going to want to have kids one day." The doctors said, "Don't worry about it. Just keep taking your meds." I explained to them that they wanted me to take one pill every 4 hours, but I'm having to take two every couple hours. I said, "I'm also having to call in sick to work. There has to be something we can do." And they said, "No, you'll be okay." I'm not blaming the physicians for my addiction, but I am saying that they contributed to it because they would not listen to me.

After 6 painful years, I was taking daily medication. I had to go shopping for a doctor who would do the surgery. I didn't care what anyone said. One night, I packed my bag and went to the emergency room. I was going to be very defiant and refuse to leave until they got my pain under control. But they wouldn't admit me. I don't know why but, God, I was so pissed. The ER doc said, "Well, we can give you a shot of morphine and send you home." I cried, "Really? That's your solution!?" I was so frustrated. I just couldn't believe it.

After I was finally able to get the surgery, I thought, "Oh, no! Now I have to be without my meds." I didn't know if I'd go through withdrawal or not, but not taking the meds made me feel like I was missing something, kind of like thinking I forgot to take my hormones. It was such a regular thing. I didn't have pounding headaches or anything. I was a little scared to go without—they were such a security blanket.

I faked a back injury so I could get physical therapy. That's when I started doing the hospital visits and physical therapy when I didn't really need them. The physical therapists couldn't understand why I was never making any progress. They said, "We have to have a goal here." But I didn't want to stop the meds. I knew as long as I had PT, I had my meds. So that was my goal, but I couldn't tell them. They really wanted to know, "What else can we do to help you?" "I don't know," I lied. I just wanted to keep the meds coming. It was terrible.

Finally, I got busted and was forced into recovery. Now everything is so much better. So much better. Things are just so much easier—waking up, going to the grocery store. I thought about the time I was high and went out and bought a car. I went out to get an oil change, and I came back having bought a new car. Crazy. But when I sobered up the next day, I cancelled the check. (I hadn't driven the new car off the lot because I had ordered it.) It didn't make the dealer too happy. Anyway, it's just amazing what a person can do under the influence.

Now things make more sense. They didn't for a while. I mean, early recovery really sucked. I would get so mad at people in the meetings who claimed to be on a pink cloud. They would say, "I haven't had a drink in weeks, and I love my life. I have so much energy, and I feel so amazing!" And I'd think, "Where in the hell is this coming from?" Because I never had the pink cloud.

Still, life is just so much easier in recovery. If you're new in recovery, suck it up and get through it. Chew your hands, eat a metal post, do whatever it takes to not get high. Just get through it. Go to a meeting. Everything will get easier.

References

Alcoholics Anonymous. (2001). *Alcoholics Anonymous,* 4th Edition. New York: A.A. World Services.

6

reentry and the return home

Most of this book deals with work-related concerns. However, one of the main obstacles to recovery may not be at work. Home-life turmoil can be a risk factor. This chapter discusses the role that home life, including family and friends, can play in your recovery. It also introduces another big issue that pertains to family and friends: codependency.

Home-Life Pressures

There is a belief that people can separate work and home into compartments, a practice called *compartmentalizing*. Yes, you can sometimes leave work issues at work and home issues at home. But to believe that chronic or significant stress in one place will not affect the other is wishful thinking. Regardless of whether you have support or strife at home, it will affect your recovery—hence this chapter's focus on stories and information for the home front.

When it comes to telling family, friends, and acquaintances about your addiction, you may encounter a mixture of responses. This is a bag that can be full of surprises—some happy, some alarming. You might reach in expecting understanding and support, only to pull out accusations and anger. Or perhaps you anticipate escaping with half your arm and come up with an armful of kindness and forgiveness instead. The best strategy is to be prepared to respond to any reaction with calm compassion.

Dan

I thought I was the only nurse who screwed up. I felt horrible. But my dad's in recovery, my wife's very understanding, as well as my wife's dad, so I've got a bunch of support around me. That's nice.

Aubrey

When I started telling people about my addiction, everyone was very loving and caring. In fact, people kept coming up with stories: "Oh yeah, I know someone who was addicted, too...." That's always the first thing they say. They tell you about somebody else they know that this happened to.

Jamie

I had to call my husband, who couldn't come and get me after my intervention because he was drunk. He's an alcoholic. So when I got home, the fight was on. It was ugly. I was not in an environment that was conducive to recovery. He drank all the time. Alcohol really wasn't my thing, but I could've crossed over easily. It was just an ugly situation for a long time.

I had to make a choice: It's either my recovery or I go crazy again. Leaving my husband was a hard decision to make. I wasn't working. I had surrendered my license. That left me the sole provider for three kids. There was a point where I had to go on food stamps, and I was damn grateful for every nickel of it. For a while, I couldn't feed my kids.

The intervention was probably the worst day and the best day of my life at the same time. I could look back at it and say that the staff conducting the intervention did all these things wrong, but in fact they propelled me into something that I needed to do, and I had known it for a long time. I got stubborn; I got defiant. My drugs were prescribed after surgery. "Are you going to tell me not to take my drugs?" I asked. But the fact of the matter is, my addiction was terrible. It was terrible. The dose kept getting bigger; the tolerance kept getting greater; there were more drugs added—it was just a mess.

A roadmap would have helped at the time. Something like, "Okay, you had a drug and alcohol evaluation saying you weren't a drug addict, but we see that you're chemically dependent. This is what you need to do: Go to rehab [and] check yourself into outpatient."

Before sharing or oversharing with family or friends, it is usually best to gather the wisdom and experience of your recovery team. For example, your 6-year-old may want to know why you have to leave him for so many meetings. Your team will help you develop an explanation that does not confuse or worry your child. No matter how rough some of your experiences at home might feel, there is help available from your recovery team and other support systems. (For more information on sharing, refer to Chapter

5, "Recovery: Getting It and Keeping It," in the section "Disclosure: Who, When, and How Much to Tell.")

Family and Friends

Just as the road to recovery is difficult for you, it is also very likely a struggle for those around you. You have expectations for your friends and family, and those expectations vary radically depending on whether you are using or you are in recovery. During your active addiction, do you remember asking your significant others to cover for you? ("Please call in sick for me today. I'm so hung over! And get off my back. I work hard to pay the bills around here. You've never had it so good!")

Now that you've entered recovery, you might expect them to be perfect recovery partners—to understand the demands of your program and give you frequent pats on the back. You may also believe you're entitled to an automatic reinstatement of trust because *this* time when you say you've turned over a new leaf, you mean it. You assume that someone who was a good enabler should now be a good recovery partner. When you were *finally* ready to make the leap, you naïvely thought your significant others would seamlessly make the shift with you.

Everyone, including those who wanted you to get help, will encounter challenges with your shifting lifestyle. Transition can be uncomfortable, if not downright painful. Standard operating procedure is no longer standard. Some things will be turned inside out. Think about a child who feels invisible and is yearning for his parent's attention. Then suddenly, Dad becomes attentive. "Gee, this is great!" the child thinks. "I got my dad back." But a few weeks later, "Dad, back off a little. I wanted your attention. I didn't want you to be in all my business." There will be awkward moments and a lot of recalibrating.

One of the major recalibrations for the family is reorienting from isolation to more social engagement. It is often an unspoken agreement to minimize or keep the addiction hidden from outsiders. Not only does the addicted person become increasingly more isolated from others as the disorder increases, the family also becomes more closed off from the world. Family members recruited in the secret conspiracy to cover for the addict also want to avoid embarrassment. Children and spouses won't invite others over for play or socializing. You never know when Mom is going to erupt into a rage, pass out on the sofa, or career off the walls. When the using, secrecy, and shame cease, and recovery begins, it is a big adjustment to see Mom building relationships outside the family with her new recovery friends.

Al

After exiting treatment, I can now look at what was going on around me, outside of my use. I didn't have any friends. I didn't communicate with my wife. I was sick. I knew I needed help, and I just wanted someone to figure out that I was using because I couldn't stop. No one I worked with ever said anything. My wife never said anything. My life was a mess before I got sober.

Brandi

While I was using, I was very isolated and never went out much. When I got sober, I had to change my whole way of life. AA helped me there. I started to socialize. I remember telling my dad, "People actually respond when I say 'Hi' and smile at them!"

"Life begins at the end of your comfort zone." I saw that on a card in a coffee shop. I said, "Yeah. I'm going to take a yoga class and have the instructor teach me how to teach yoga. I'm going to go for it."

I got a job at the gym doing personal training. I taught yoga, which was really uncomfortable at first, as I don't like getting up in front of people. That was a big breakthrough. I did it on purpose, knowing that it would help me get out of isolating. Stepping out like that helped a lot.

Obviously, you need support from recovery friends and counselors, but the entire family needs support as well. Substance use disorder (SUD) is a disease of isolation and fear. Fear is often a driving emotion not only for you, but also for your family members, who are facing a lot of uncertainty and change. Family members may be asking, "What about me? I didn't ask for this. What will happen to our lives? Our home?" Anger is often a symptom of underlying fears. "How could you do this to me? Why didn't you tell me? I thought things were supposed to get better, not worse!" Frustration, confusion, and feelings of helplessness abound. "If I couldn't admit to myself I had a problem, how could I tell my husband?"

According to a national poll conducted by the Hazelden Foundation (2008), alcohol and drug abuse or addiction affects all within the family, not just the afflicted individual. Also, 36 percent of employees admitted that at least one of their coworkers had been distracted, was less productive, or missed work because of SUD within their family.

Conflicts arise with partners, children, friends, and finances. Some will be lucky and start with a good support system. For other family members, it will take time to rebuild trust and become more educated about living with someone in recovery. Some of you will never have a good family support system. Even so, you are not alone. You will have a sponsor, a support group, and access to a rich community through Alcoholics Anonymous/ Narcotics Anonymous (AA/NA) and other recovery groups.

The good news is, if you are sincere about recovery, there is always good news! As the preceding testimonies relate, the process might feel anything but pleasant, but the outcomes will turn your life around.

Codependency

Codependence is a common thread among family, friends, and addicts. *Codependence* creates and nurtures the environment for addiction. Codependence refers to the unhealthy relationship between an alcoholic/ addict and his or her partner. Codependence is often used to describe enabling actions, a lack of self-esteem, and an unhealthy need to "fix" another person, thereby abandoning one's own needs and identity. A dominant codependency trait is overruling a healthy boundary to accommodate someone else's unhealthy behavior. As mentioned, codependency originally referred to partners of addicts. After the using stops, it gets easier to spot the codependent nature in addicts as well.

When looking at codependency, consider these areas: traits or behaviors of the addict/alcoholic and traits or behaviors of the significant other(s). Nurses are notorious for placing others' needs before their own. How often do you hear about the nurse who didn't take her lunch break or who "forgot" to use the restroom? Who stayed 16 hours instead of 12? Have you gone to work with cold symptoms because "Who will care for the patient if I don't show up?"

In the 1970s, counselors who treated alcoholics and their families identified common behaviors that enabled the alcoholic to continue using. For example, children in an alcoholic situation will often take on a parental role, becoming responsible for their using parent. Where there are addicts, there are enablers. Enablers protect addicts from their consequences. That allows the enabler to feel needed and to feel a measure of control in a chaotic environment. They say, "I have to help him. What if he becomes homeless?" Or, "What if the neighbors find out my son is an addict?" Or, "What if she loses her job? I can't afford to support her." Even though the addict is the identified patient, with a sick version of support (codependent family), family members can enable the patient to death!

As an addict's relative or coworker, it is important to remember that you are *not* the cause of their using problem. You cannot cure it, nor can you control it. However, you must realize that you may be contributing to the user's problem.

NOTE *Although this discussion of enabling may appear as though it is directed at someone other than the addict, it is included in this book so the addict can become aware of the enabler's role in his or her addiction.*

Most addicts are fraught with codependent traits. If not recognized and addressed at some point, these traits stunt recovery. You don't have to figure this out in early recovery; that comes later with treatment and working steps with sponsors and counselors. However, it is good to understand that when you peel back the layers of active use, you likely will find your own codependence beneath it all.

Here are some examples of enabling behaviors (Morrow, n.d.):

> Giving money to someone to spend on drink or drugs
> Engaging in arguments with an addict, knowing that he or she will use it as an excuse to use or drink
> Doing the addict's dirty work for him or her—for example, calling the user's boss to say he or she is sick and can't come to work
> Making excuses for his or her using ("He's under a lot of stress.")
> Accepting the user's excuses ("I'm under a lot of stress.")
> Using with the addict/alcoholic
> Always having drugs in the house
> Giving the user drugs or alcohol because it puts him or her in a good mood
> Always trying to "fix" the user
> Always giving the user "one more chance"…and then another…oh yes, and another…and so it goes on
> Pretending the user doesn't have a problem, and the behavior is normal and acceptable
> Taking on jobs or chores that the addict should be doing

Author Tian Dayton notes:

> It is critical that all members of a nurse's family or support system get help to cope with the negative feelings and destructive behaviors that characterize the person with a substance use

disorder. A critical component to good recovery is emotional sobriety, which is defined as finding and maintaining our equilibrium. The essence of emotional sobriety is good self-regulation. Self-regulation means that we have mastered those skills that allow us to balance our moods, our nervous systems, our appetites, our sexual drive, and our sleep. We have learned how to tolerate our intense emotions without acting out in dysfunctional ways by clamping down or foreclosing on our feeling world or self-medicating (Dayton, 2007, p. 3).

Members of a family with an addict in their midst often take on different roles, including the following (Missouri Department of Social Services, 2006):

> **The chemically dependent:** This person experiences a progression of guilt, shame, and growing fear. He or she denies the problem by hiding it behind a wall of defense and remaining basically an adolescent in terms of emotional growth. This false front gives others in the family the illusion that the chemically dependent person is okay.

> **The chief enabler:** This person is closest to the chemically dependent and is the one on whom the chemically dependent most relies for his or her self-worth. The chief enabler is inevitably affected by the user's mood swings. To keep a facade of normalcy, the chief enabler becomes more and more responsible for perpetuating the facade.

> **The family hero:** This is usually, but not always, the oldest child. This person sees and hears more of what is happening in the family unit. The family hero feels responsible for the pain and turmoil in the family and works hard to make things better. This person often excels in academics, sports, or social organizations and brings favorable recognition to himself or herself and the family. He or she may appear quite mature, responsible, and healthy. However, hidden beneath the surface are loneliness, guilt, fear, and anger.

> **The scapegoat:** Usually identified by the family as "the problem," this person is usually the second child. He or she is quite often deprived of positive attention, which is given to the hero, and deprived of the immense energy that the chemically dependent may require. Quite often cute, humorous, and fragile, sometimes loud and precocious, the scapegoat gets attention in negative ways through disruptive behavior. Few outsiders see the fear and insecurity within the child. Scapegoats are often blamed for many of the family problems, which are not their fault. "You would drink, too, if you had a child like that," is often heard about the scapegoat. The scapegoat comes to act in a manner that will justify the accusations and often develops substance-abuse problems himself or herself.

> **The lost child:** This child tends to be withdrawn—a loner whose most valuable contribution is that he or she does not disrupt or demand attention. Because the family's attention is focused elsewhere, there is little attention available anyway. The lost child suffers loneliness, even though loneliness is most comfortable for them. As family turmoil increases, the lost child often finds validation in fantasy. Without help, it is almost impossible to find this validation in himself or herself, resulting in low self-esteem. The lost child stands a good chance of becoming depressed and addicted to alcohol or drugs or becoming an adult involved in codependency situations.

> **The mascot:** This is usually the family clown—the one who will do virtually anything to make other family members feel better. Mascots take on the job of relieving tension and lessening crisis. They are very sensitive to the moods and needs of others. When mascots reach adulthood, they have trouble recognizing and meeting their own needs and dealing with stress.

In looking at both sides of codependency, can you recognize yourself? Have you been the martyr in your workplace? Are you an enabler in your home life? The takeaway for you is this: You do not have to fix everything now. You don't have to fix the family or solve all concerns at your job. You just have to stay clean and sober. Increase your awareness. Become curious about your own codependent dynamics. Learn to set boundaries. A codependent can find help in Al-Anon. There are many helpful books and CDs on codependency; see Appendix E, "Supporting Materials" for examples. Counseling can be of great service. Sharing in a support group can help identify your blind spots.

VOICES

If you begin the process of recovery, there is the possibility of greater self-awareness and greater boundaries. And that doesn't just mean saying no; that means being comfortable with allowing other people and patients to be who they are. So you don't get mad at the man who's dying. And you don't necessarily get upset with the drug addict and cause conflicts that don't need to be. I think you get to be a more compassionate nurse. I think you get, in some respects, a more caring nurse or somebody who's able to care properly and express it appropriately. That is opposed to caring, because "I need to feel good about me, and you getting better makes me feel better about me."

Recovering nurses will come to know the difference between empathy and sympathy. That has to do with boundaries again. That makes them a better nurse. As a patient, I would much rather have an empathetic nurse who can intuit what's going on and take appropriate actions as opposed to someone who is just as reactive to my emotional state, and we're both a basket case as I lie there in the bed being anxious.

–Mark H. Broadhead, MD

Gina

I can just hear my mother saying, "Well, we don't have any addicts in our family. It must be [my husband's] fault that you're an addict." And still to this day, their relationship is very strained, even though he has been in recovery too and doing well.

Last week, my daughter got into some trouble stealing, and I know she's using. The point is, now I can see her in a different perspective. My parents saw it from one perspective, but because I've been through it, I can look at her through different eyes. I don't have to be so critical. I can be of service. I can be there when she needs me, without rescuing her.

I'm actually grateful I've been through this. When it comes to being a parent and having children with a problem, I'm grateful I understand. I think of how my parents and dad's parents treated addiction. Before his recovery, my dad acted like I'd cut his arms and legs off. I had done this horrendous thing to him. I don't have any legal problems or anything, but he thought it was terrible what I had done to him. Thank goodness I'm stopping the cycle of judgment with my children.

Lena's Story

The first time I got caught diverting, I denied it but jumped through the hoops. I did what they told me, sponsored myself, and stayed clean and sober for 8 years. That was 5 years in the BON program and then 3 years after. Then my life started spinning out of control financially. I went berserk with money. I quit paying attention to my checkbook. I wasn't using yet, but I wasn't balancing my checkbook and I wasn't making payments. Then I was overdrafting; I couldn't keep up with all of it. I started using, calling in prescriptions, something I said I would never ever do.

I don't remember the first time I called in, but I remember where I was when I did it. I was working on the chemical dependency unit. I had hurt my back and continued getting refills. They wanted me to have surgery, and I didn't want to go that route. The surgeon quit calling in for me, so I started calling them in using two of the doctors I work with. I called them in for me, my family, my parents who live in another state using their names. I had everybody's information and birthdate.

I got caught when the pharmacy called my daughter and told her that she could get her medications more cheaply if she went through mail order. She said to the pharmacist, "I don't even know what you're talking about because I'm not taking any meds." That prompted the pharmacist to call work. He said from January to that time, I would have accumulated 25 felonies. I think it probably would've been more, but he said 25. The pharmacist really, really wanted to press charges. He called the DNS and voiced his concerns. He wanted to pursue charges and wanted to talk to the two doctors who were used to call in the scripts.

I was at court the day I got the call. I had gotten a ticket for inattentive driving (I'm sure it was because of meds), and I wasn't feeling good (detox). My DNS had left several hysterical messages on my phone. It was the start of my kids' spring break, so they were home. They heard it. When I called Mary, my DNS at the time, my husband and kids were right there and they knew. So it was all out, "Yeah, I've been taking all these meds again."

I went to the state board first and turned in my license. In the meantime, my DNS was in the process of calling sister facilities, trying to find some place for me to go to detox. She knew I was not going to be doing well. She scheduled me a flight, got me a ticket, and told me that I was going to Las Vegas. I thought that was bizarre because most people go to Vegas to party, but I was going there to sober up. She said, "If we don't take care of our own, then we have no business being here. That is what we do here." She worked in chemical dependency and had dealt with a daughter who had a meth addiction. So she knew.

My flight wasn't supposed to leave until later that night. I was at home devastated. My whole life was in turmoil. I was crying hysterically. I couldn't believe that I had done this again. I knew it, but I couldn't believe it. In the meantime, the pharmacist had called the two doctors to urge them to press charges. They said, "Absolutely not, we will not charge her. She's a fabulous nurse, and we're going to do what we can to help." My program manager had called me and thought there might be a chance that I could be arrested if the pharmacy kept pursuing it. I was at home waiting. I was totally terrified because I'd never been arrested before, ever. Finally, I flew to Vegas.

The first few days in inpatient, I was so sick that I was in bed. When I finally started coming around, I remember telling myself, "Okay, Lena, you're a patient. You don't know anything." Obviously, I didn't know anything about recovery. It hadn't yet worked for me. So I was trying to be a perfect patient. I'd go to meals, I'd go to groups. I listened to all the information. I went to counseling. They medically stabilized me and detoxed me. But I was still was pretty sick when I got home.

After I got back, the realization of going through the whole 5-year program again hit me. I thought that I was handling things right, but I was hostile. Not at anybody else, but at me. I was angry beyond belief that I had done this again to myself and my family. I kept pushing my monitor to get my license back. I would ask my monitor, "What else do you want? I went through a 28-day program. I'm better! I'm better!"

I wasn't better. I was detoxed, but I wasn't better. I just wanted my license back so I could get back to work. "Yes I'll go to these meetings and I'll pay this money and I'll do this and that, but I can't if I don't have my license because I can't make the money. I'm the only support in my house." My husband wasn't working. So I fought it and fought it. I demanded meetings with the monitoring director, John. He met with me.

John wouldn't tell me anything except "Keep doing what you're doing." I didn't know what that meant. I was going to the meetings, people were signing my slips, I had a sponsor already. I was doing the urine tests. "What do you mean keep doing what I'm doing? You guys aren't doing anything back for me." I was pissed. So I fought it and fought it.

My sponsor kept telling me, "You need to chill out. You need to get on your hands and knees and pray." I thought I was praying. And I kept asking my higher power to help me. Well, that wasn't what I needed to be doing. What I needed to do was to surrender everything to my higher power and admit that I could not handle this. I prayed, "I need you to take it from me and do what you will with it because I can't do it. I can't do it." And I remember being on my hands and knees and sobbing. But when I was done, I was so refreshed, like being baptized again. I felt clean, like I could breathe. There was a sense of peace that came over me. From that point on, things just started getting better.

I remember going to a nurse support meeting and the facilitator said, "Oh, my God." He could see the change in me. I remember going to an AA meeting, and one guy said, "It warms my heart so much when I've watched somebody struggle and struggle and then one day, the lights come on." From that point on, things just started clicking. I totally did what my sponsor told me to do. If she had told me to run around naked in a parking lot, I would've done it.

I found my sponsor. I had seen her occasionally, in my meetings. Just listening to her, I knew that I needed her. Her story wasn't like mine. Her drug of choice is alcohol. But she grew up in an alcoholic home like I did. I understood what she was saying, and I knew she was right for me. I knew that she wouldn't be easy on me. I'd had a few sponsors before her, and I obviously wasn't ready for them. I did what they told me to do, but…. I told her, "I don't want you to be easy on me. I was too easy on myself when I sponsored myself and look where it got me."

After about a year, I got my license back. In that year, I was doing my outpatient treatment, and my company let me stay as a psych tech, comparable to working as a CNA. They paid me better than they pay psych techs, but it wasn't even close to what I was used to making as an RN. Even though it was humbling, it was wonderful to be so cared for.

Working as a psych tech was a step down. I had been the house supervisor. I discussed with my DNS how to approach the staff. We could have a staff meeting, put out a memo, or just not address it. She left the choice to me but said, "Here's the bottom line. If people treat you badly,

I want to know. Not that they're going to be in trouble, but they need to be counseled." I decided I would just deal with people as the issue came up. If they asked me, I would tell them. Eventually, everybody I worked with closely knew about my situation.

Some of my friends at work had buffered my return. I had asked them to say that I was having a problem with substances. I was getting some treatment and I would be back, although I probably wouldn't be back in a nursing position for a while. So a lot of that was already done for me. It still didn't make it easy to come back, though.

My DNS did not have to counsel anyone. There was one nurse who didn't want me back working, but I thought, "Okay, I don't need to talk to her anymore. I don't need to associate with people who are going to make me feel bad about all of this." So it all worked out.

I went to an outpatient treatment program. I loved outpatient, more than inpatient. I think inpatient is just a glimmer into recovery. Outpatient really helped me find out who I am. I did see a lot of people who were only there because they were ordered by the courts. But my core group had several other nurses who were also in the recovery program. There was also a lawyer and a policeman's daughter. We were there because we wanted to save our lives, save our families, and keep our jobs.

When I first got sober, my job was my main focus. I thought, "Oh, my God. I can't pay my bills. How can I pay for treatment?" It seemed impossible, but I did it. I figured it out. You may have to get rid of the cable TV; you may have to quit doing some extra activities. You have to cut back if you want to live. That might be what you have to do to make it. And then recovery gets easier, and the rest is history.

I have stayed in contact with my sponsor on a weekly basis. If things get tough, I call her more than once a week. I go to AA; I do my steps. I can pick out when I'm having relapse behaviors. I'll call my sponsor and say, "Is that a behavior?" And she'll say, "Well, do you think it's a relapse behavior?" "Absolutely," I'll say. And she'll say, "Then do some steps on it. We'll talk about it." I never would have even looked at my behavior before, much less asked someone else's opinion of it. So I think I've grown a thousand times.

I've gotten closer to my husband. When all this started to come down, I didn't think we would be able to stay together. I figured I had damaged him and broken our relationship enough. He has changed too. He was enabling me before, but he didn't recognize it as that. My whole family will call me on my crap now if I'm out of line. Sometimes this journey gets frustrating, but I'm only 5 years into it and it gets easier, 1 day at a time.

I have a lot to offer now that I'm sober. I have stories to tell. I share stories with some patients who I think are ready to hear them and maybe are looking for a glimmer of hope. Like Liz, another woman in nurse support group. I talked to her because she didn't know anything about the PRN program. I rushed out to visit her (in detox) and told her, "There is a program for you." I remember her asking, "Will I ever be able to work as a nurse?" I replied, "Yes, you will work as a nurse." I've since seen her. She had come full circle by the time she came to our nurse meetings. I don't think I have been hugged as tight by a person as she hugged me when I told her, "There's a program for us." The nursing community doesn't talk about PRN. They don't let nurses know that there's a program.

You may ask, what has worked for me this time? I need to stay in contact; I need to keep going to meetings; I need to stay with my sponsor; I need to be accountable to my family, to my coworkers, and to me. As far as I'm concerned, the PRN program saved my life! I was bitter and angry, as bitter as many are when they first get into this program and have to sign that contract. It seems so overwhelming. But it saved my life, and it saved my family. Thank God the state board is willing to work with and help us through this because some states' boards of nursing don't.

References

Dayton, T. (2007). *Emotional sobriety: From relationship trauma to resilience and balance.* Deerfield Beach, FL: HCI Books.

Hazelden Foundation. (2008). Family substance abuse affects American workers. Retrieved from http://alcoholism.about.com/od/work/a/blhaz050331.htm

Kuntsche, S., Knibbe, R. A., & Gmel, G. (2009). Social roles and alcohol consumption: a study of 10 industrialised countries. *Soc Sci Med, 68,* 1263–70.

Missouri Department of Social Services. (2006). Substance abuse—Recovery resources. *Child Welfare Manual.* Retrieved from http://www.dss.mo.gov/cd/info/cwmanual/section7/ch1_33/sec7ch16.htm

Morrow, D. (n.d.). Enabling an alcoholic. *The Alcoholism Guide.* Retrieved from http://www.the-alcoholism-guide.org/enabling-an-alcoholic.htm

7

careers and change

It may feel as though you've lost everything when you begin recovery. For some, nursing is a vocation that involves a great investment. For others, it may be an avocation. Either way, if you're invested in your identity as a nurse, it can feel surreal or devastating to have this identity in question. This chapter addresses the discomfort of identity loss and shifting into a new professional paradigm. In addition, it covers employment options and early-recovery considerations.

Adjusting: The Mental/Emotional Transition

You probably take pride in being a nurse. Losing your nursing identity could feel like losing a huge chunk of yourself. Your self-esteem, status, and reputation are up for review. It wouldn't be unusual to feel threatened, lost, confused, appalled, scared, resentful, or...fill in the blank. What are you feeling? Whatever it is, you don't have to use to cover up those feelings.

While your emotions can be overwhelming, if you let them move through you, they will eventually subside. When you get on the other side of the storm, you will realize more and more that you won't die. They are just feelings. They're not even reality. They can feel real, but they aren't anything but emotion. And contrary to popular opinion, emotion isn't fatal. Emotion doesn't kill us; it's our inability to cope that does.

Employing good recovery tools will give you options and, eventually, freedom from compulsion. How do you break through a trance? Someone or something has to snap you out of it. Do something to break the spell. Do the opposite of what you're used to doing. Do the opposite of what you *think* you feel like doing. Snap to! You've been brainwashed. Addiction is the worst kind of cult you can join. Your head and your cells scream, "Do it! Follow that leader! You have no choice!" You blindly break every vow you've made to yourself and others to stay in this cult. It's time to break the spell.

You never have to drink or use again. Part of intentional recovery is finding out what has burst the spell of addiction for millions. For example, many have learned tools and developed support to deal with feelings and cravings. It is common to hear in support groups, "I used to use to change the way they felt; now, I change the way I feel, and I don't have to use." The list of tools to change your focus and your feelings is long.

For more tools and resources, see Chapter 5, "Recovery: Getting It and Keeping It."

NOTE

Moving from addictive thinking to recovery thinking swaps a negative focus for a positive perspective. It is easy to mourn all the health, time, money, relationships, promotions, and material things lost. That type of thinking, however, is first-rate justification for relapsing. Shifting focus to how much there is to be grateful for and what you have to build from is first-rate recovery thinking. This doesn't mean you can't grieve the losses, but it does mean that you also appreciate what is good in your life. Begin now. Take 10 minutes and make a list of 20 things you still have going for you. You don't have to be overly specific. Add in any asset. This list will come in handy later when you are feeling stuck and hopeless or interviewing for a job. Here a few ideas to start your list:

> Education
> Experience (how many years, in what areas)
> Positive attitude
> Supportive manager
> Skilled in a crisis
> Resiliency
> Problem-solving skills
> Ability to innovate

It bears repeating that whether you feel overwhelmed and lost now or in the future, this list-making is an important tool to shift focus from what isn't working into a field of positivity and possibility. Later, we will look at how list-making applies to job hunting as well.

The Three Amigos: Denial, Ego, and Control

Working to derail your recovery are the three amigos: denial, ego, and control.

Denial

If you aren't already well-acquainted with denial, let us introduce you to one of the main actors in your drama. It's the first character you might wrestle with in recovery and career matters. As mentioned in Chapter 5, denial is the overlord of addiction. It's a slick talker trying to sell you a deadly bargain. Harboring denial is like making a deal with the devil.

You know how the story goes: The hero is seduced into thinking he's getting some great boon for next to nothing. All he has to do is sign on the dotted line. He goes through his days until, at some unexpected moment, payment comes due—and it's terrifying. Keep this character in mind. Denial can crop up anytime in an addict's life, and it's a carrier of the disease.

Karen

For the first 3 months in my outpatient treatment program, I sat with my arms folded across my chest. I was thinking, "When I'm done with this program, I'm going to have my glass of wine. I got here because of my addiction to opiates. My problem was never alcohol." During the course of treatment, however, I changed my take on the matter. First, I didn't want to drink anymore. I heard in treatment, "You only drink to change the way you feel." I no longer feel the need to change the way I feel! And I don't choose to have the consequences that could come with that drink. I thought my problem was only opiates. With the education I received in my treatment program, I realized a drug is a drug is a drug.

Ego

There is a lot of fuel for the ego in nursing. Note how special you are. You belong to a special population with special knowledge, including the following:

> Lifesaving skills
> An uncommon coded language
> Pharmacological knowledge
> Ingesting and injecting medicine as the norm
> The ability to take charge
> The ability to act as an authority figure
> Professional detachment
> Comfort with needles
> Self-diagnoses

Eureka! That's a volatile formula: denial with a superiority complex! This doesn't necessarily apply to you, but it might. Some drug/alcohol counselors have identified the nursing ego and smug defense mechanisms as huge obstacles to rehabilitation. The caution here is if you find yourself automatically resorting to "knowing more than others, and therefore knowing better," that kind of thinking is worth evaluating.

You can pick your ego or your life. Ego-laced denial can range from a flat-out "I don't have a problem" to a bargain that sounds like "Yes, I have a problem with opiates, but drinking was never an issue." This is when you hold out that you are not a person with an addictive nature. You believe that you are special and that you are exempt from cross-addiction. It's a theory that many have unsuccessfully put to the test.

Kim

Why did I get a job selling phones in early recovery? I wouldn't have answered then as I will now. When I first got into the program, I was cocky. I took that job only because I had to. I looked at selling phones as more humiliating than humbling. I had to show "them" that I wasn't all the way down. I had something to prove. Now I know it was my ego. I never thought I had a big ego, as I was always doing for others. It has taken a long time for me to realize and admit that my ego has been in the way. It's all so clear to me now. It was more humiliating than humbling at the time because I didn't learn from it. To be humbled, you gain wisdom. To feel humiliation is more from fear, anger, and self-pity.

Control

Why talk about ego, denial, and control when discussing careers? It is a huge impulse to want to control your destiny by immediately being re-instated or re-creating the job/position/role that just disintegrated due to your substance abuse. Like a salmon swimming back upstream, it feels natural to return home to your old comfort zone. Not only that, but you have denial and its buddy, ego, telling you that it's just fine for you to return to work without giving it a second thought. There's a classic progression that sounds like this: I'm caught. I'm lost. I'm repentant. I'm renewed. I'm ready to return to my previous position. I've got this under control.

Nothing could be further from the truth. If after 60 days, 6 months, or 1 year of being clean and sober, you think you're ready to return to the circumstances that got you here, be cautious. You may think you have it under control because you haven't used for a few days, but that is nothing like being back in a zone of strain and seduction.

Annie

I was only sober for 3 months when I got pregnant. That's when I was selling meat off the back of a truck, pregnant. I had no license. I couldn't find a job. I saw an ad in the paper and went to work for people selling meat off the back of a truck. I had gotten pregnant that January and I remember thinking how grateful I was that I wasn't using, because I don't think I could've stopped.

Questions to Ask Yourself

True or false:

> I want to get clean and sober so I can get my job back.
> I want to get a job that supports my recovery.
> I want to say "Yes, I'm fine," as soon as possible.
> I want to think things through so that I'm more confident that I will maintain my sobriety and not endanger myself and others.

These questions are reflections of how thoroughly you have thought through your impulse and desire to get back to work. Are you operating on autopilot, flying a preprogrammed course that can take you right back into another crash? Or are you thinking through the course ahead, including all the inherent hazards and safeguards?

Aside from the logistical issues of when and where you can work, there's also the question of self-preparedness. This is a question of maturity, wisdom, and dedication to your long-term best interests. It's a case of, "If I can keep my job, or if I can get hired for a different job, should I accept?" In other words, will this job be a good fit for your recovery and, therefore, for you? There are a few negative motivators for wanting to get a job or retain an old position; while it might be possible, is it positive?

Most people can conjure memories of "having to have it" to the point of missing the bigger picture. Think of a young bride lost in the fantasy of her dream wedding, failing to realize what the lifelong marriage entails.

When considering a position, be prepared to answer these questions:

> Why do I want this position? What are my real motives? Is it because it's the only work I know and it's in my comfort zone? Is it because I have something to atone for or to prove to my old colleagues?

> What should I be concerned about in this job environment? What's the emotional load?

> What triggers that have created cravings/obsession/compulsion for using in the past are present in this environment?

> Do I have sober/recovery support in this environment? If not, can I get some? Either way, how do I go in forearmed? What are my strategies and tools (my instead-of-using list)? For instance, what should I say when offered a narcotic pain med? Am I prepared to leave if I feel a craving? What can I do to feel grounded, fed, and rested versus H.A.L.T. (hungry, angry, lonely, and tired)? What can I do to be mentally and spiritually fit? Am I prepared to handle adverse conversations, attitudes, confrontations, and criticism?

> How long have I been clean/sober/in recovery?

> What are my new coping skills for stress?

> Will this job make it difficult to access my recovery program? Will it interfere with meetings and appointments?

> Have I discussed my motives and the ramifications of this job with my sponsor, peer support group, and others in recovery?

NOTE | *Don't want to be bothered with this? Think your love and passion for the work will carry you through? Think again.*

> Am I in a hurry to cover up all my past mistakes and make everything right, as fast as possible?

> Do I think I have recovered from all and any temptation to use again, am bulletproof, and am invincible due to my great intellect, moral character, and supreme willpower? In other words, I have fully repented and am now saved from my old sinful past. I shall not sin against myself, my coworkers, my patients, or society. I have done penance and am born again.

Career Considerations

You have a number of career choices to make. These choices are contingent on circumstances, including licensing as well as mental, emotional, and physical concerns.

With respect to licensing, your circumstances may be any of the following:

> You are still employed as a nurse.

> You are still employed as a nurse with restrictions.

> Your license has been suspended.

> Your license has been revoked. (Note that this affects licensing in other states. For more information, refer to Chapter 3, "Getting Back to Work," in the section "Treatment and Monitoring Contracts for Licensing.")

> You still have your license.

> You still have your license, but you just got fired.

Your mental, emotional, and physical concerns might include the following:

> You want to continue nursing and keep it business as usual. In that case, look out for sensory stimulants such as sights, sounds, smells, and tastes that translate into triggers/cravings/compulsions. In

addition, home, work, and global (politics, world affairs, economic) stressors are a concern, as are the attitudes of your coworkers, managers, patients, family, friends, associates (church, school, peer groups), and yourself.

> Your return to nursing is delayed, deferred, or interrupted. For example, nursing is postponed until you feel more established in recovery or your license is reinstated. You may also have a pending sentence to serve in jail, prison, or work release (with restricted hours). Or, it could be that you want to nurse but in a different capacity or environment.

> You want to change careers. Maybe you are no longer physically capable of nursing, or maybe you simply no longer want to be a nurse.

Most nurses take a temporary voluntary or mandatory sabbatical from nursing. Of course, circumstances vary from wanting to leave nursing and being forced to leave. (More on those distinctions in a moment.) Right now, the mental chatter you hear might sound like, "What do I do now?", "What's going to happen to me?", and "What's going to happen to my family?"

The chatter can continue on and on and sound like the following:

> I'm scared. I'm not trained for anything else.
> I'm the breadwinner.
> What will my family do?
> How will I pay the bills?
> What if I lose the house?
> How will I feed my kids, the dog, myself?

Fears may be reflexive or recognizable. *Reflexive* fears are those our psyches have lugged around most of our lives. We haul around a special closet where these phantoms live, ready to appear when we're facing change and the unknown. Ironically, the phantoms can loom larger when we are moving in a positive direction. The more fear you have, the more likely you're closer to getting better. Think about it: Which felt scarier—the day-to-day risk of getting caught, or being asked to change in ways that are life-enhancing and lifesaving? Which option has a scarier outcome?

The second set of fears, *recognizable* fears, are attached to real considerations. They generally relate to lifestyle issues: fearing not earning enough money to keep up with your car payment, to send your child to band camp, or to fly to your granddaughter's christening. You might be gripped in panic that you will have to sell everything and move into a shelter next week. Or perhaps you're more concerned about continuing your child's piano lessons. Whatever the case, slow down, exhale slowly to counter anxiety, and make a plan to make a plan. As advised in Alcoholics Anonymous, do the next indicated thing. Get counsel from your recovery team to get clarity and empowerment.

Financial Strategies

These tips may help you build the bridge between now and your next job:

> Know your options and restrictions.

> Don't guess or make assumptions about how good or bad your financial situation is. Living in fear without doing real research is not the same as taking responsible action. Slow down and have someone on your recovery team or a financial planner help you get a clear picture of your options.

> Know your resources. These include unemployment benefits, savings, temporary employment, EAP, and so on.

> Lighten your budget. Cut expenses by carpooling, taking the city bus, stopping water deliveries, using out-of-the-box hair color, home-brewing your coffee, shopping at thrift stores, traveling closer to home, cutting cable/phone plans, etc.

> Work on finding temporary part-time or full-time employment.

> Polish your résumé and interview skills. This might include doing a strength assessment, which you can use in your cover letter and for interviews. You can work with a career coach (or use online resources), learn how to network (get your elevator speech down), and study interview techniques and role-play. Consider exploring options inside and outside your profession.

> Do the next indicated thing.

The Big Questions

At this stage, you must ask yourself two main questions. The answers determine your next course of action.

> Do I need to generate income?

> What do I want to do with the rest of my life?

If the answer to the first question is no, skip to the next question. If the answer to the first question is yes, ask yourself "How soon?" One response is fear based: "Now! I need income now! I can't wait another minute. I'm so stressed out. I'm freaking! I need another paycheck right now so that I don't have to live out of my comfort zone." Another type of response is more rational and based on concrete information. This is part of making a real plan based on real information with respect to budgeting and resources, including unemployment benefits, savings, and IRA. (Yes, recovering from a life-threatening condition counts as an emergency.)

Income Options

Build a plan. This bridge might be a temporary job in or outside a medical-related field. Here's what you need to consider:

> **Constancy:** Do you have the option to continue work with your current employer?

> **Budget:** How much do you need to continue living at your current lifestyle? Could you cut your budget and live more frugally for the interim?

> **Part time or full time:** Can you reduce your expenses and get by with a part-time position? Some advantages of working part time in early recovery include more time for treatment activities, reduced workplace stress, and reduced access to substances (depending on the work environment). If you work full time, can you select a recovery-supportive schedule and staff?

> **Nursing and/or related fields:** What are the options for nursing or nursing-related jobs? What other considerations are there? What are your fields of interest? What job listings have you seen—newspaper ads, Monster, Craigslist.org, Dice.com? What leads have you found by networking with friends, family, and associates?

With regard to what you want to do with the rest of your life, you have two choices:

> Live a life of recovery.

> Get by the best you can with diminishing mental, physical, financial, social, and emotional options.

If you choose the first option, work becomes a matter of engagement. Ask yourself what type of work will be meaningful, fulfilling, and enjoyable. This kind of work is typically characterized by the following:

> Time flies by.
> You're excited, not drained, at the end of the day.
> You light up when you talk about work.

Will nursing give this to you? Is it time to find another area of nursing? Maybe you're ready to open up to other possibilities. Although you might come back to nursing when you get your feet under you, this is a great time to examine what you would love to spend your time doing.

Maybe you don't need to work at all. In that case, decide what hobbies, groups, crafts, volunteer efforts, and other endeavors make you feel alive. What are the things that you used to love that you can reincorporate into your life? Those self-care items that slipped away—taking walks, reading, writing, painting, traveling, taking baths, cooking—will complement your recovery.

To review:

1. Plan to make a plan with your recovery team.
2. Make the plan. Include concrete (including financial) information, job options, job-hunting tools, strong strategies for staying clean and sober, and strong strategies for a recovery lifestyle.

On the Job Hunt: Tips from a Positivity Coach

Obviously, with job loss, not only is there an identity crisis, there is also financial pressure. When paychecks stop, survival instincts kick into overdrive. Most people want to resolve unemployment immediately. In early recovery, however, it is usually not permitted nor advisable to re-create your old job. Instead of job hunting like a crazy person, put your health first and take stock of your options. You are setting the foundation for a life of recovery and a new journey in your career. To begin a journey, there is nothing better than a good guidebook, compass, and map. Good news! You can find multitudes of career help online and in books.

A great affordable resource is the Positivity Academy. The Positivity Academy (www.positivityacademy.com) offers the following:

> New ways of looking at the world—at your life and opportunities—and at how to achieve lasting happiness
> Modules and tools to discover and activate your unique strengths to create a more meaningful, fulfilling, and enjoyable life

"In Pursuit of Career Fulfillment" (Morgan, 2013), Module 6 of the academy's *Unalienable Pursuits* series, offers suggestions for résumé building, interviewing, and other considerations in this job market. This module deals with five different targets:

> Getting a job
> Increasing job satisfaction
> Getting a promotion
> Promoting your own enterprise
> Transitioning into an avocation and finding meaning in retirement

According to the Positivity Academy, getting a new job mostly comes down to selling. Your very first customer is the person in the mirror. Are you worth investing in your own development? It isn't a matter of being cut out for a certain job. It is about grooming yourself to be successful. The rest of this section contains excerpts (with modifications) from the section on getting a new job.

Fate doesn't cut it. Look inward and work with your many talents, attributes, and potential to learn new things. What it takes to do a job is not what it takes to get a job. Put your energy into what it takes to land the job you want. For example, presidents are not necessarily elected for their executive abilities. They may be elected because of good marketing and promise.

One of the biggest hurdles is giving up whatever prevents you from getting what you want. What are the chains that retard your progress? What can you give up that will make space for positive growth?

A person's career is the variable most highly correlated with well-being. Elements that contribute to one's career well-being include the following:

> Having a deep purpose in life
> Using your strengths every day
> Taking opportunities to develop your innate talents
> Focusing on objectives outside your comfort zone, or stretch objectives
> A written plan to reach your goals

How you spend your time shapes your identity. High scores on career well-being double the possibility that you are thriving overall. Over time, low career well-being will take its toll and drag you down. People tend to recover more rapidly from the death of a spouse than from sustained unemployment. *Career thriving* is when you love your work and it spills over into your personal life.

Aubrey

All I've known is caregiving and nursing, so I didn't know what it was like to have a nonstressful job. I thought that was just what working is. You work, then you recover from work, and then you just gear up to go to work and you work some more. I just thought that's how it was supposed to be. I never understood people who went to 9-to-5 jobs and carried their coffee cup around and chitchatted with people in the office. I never understood people like that. But now that I'm home, I realize that I was way overstressed. I was bottling things up and not coping well at all. I enjoy my family way more. I enjoy my kids so much more. I don't get frustrated, and I'm able to live in the moment. It's nice just being at home.

Prescription for Career Development

When it comes to preparing yourself for a new job or career, it makes sense to build from your interests and your assets. Who would you rather spend 40 hours a week with? Someone who is contented and flourishing or someone who is discontented and struggling? If you've never put much thought to your interests and assets, you can increase your self-awareness by creating a master list of attributes and assets. Remember the power of list-making? Try the following:

1. Take one or more strengths assessments (DISC, StrengthsFinder, etc.).

2. Ask five or 10 friends or family members to write 20 adjectives to describe you. Alternatively, you can print a list of personality adjectives from the Internet and ask them to select 20 adjectives from the list.

3. Write down things that interest you, and then list the common traits.

4. Recall what people say when they compliment you. For example, "You're always so curious and ask the best questions. You really get us thinking."

As you become more aware and intentional about living from your strengths and interests, you can find ways to activate them every day. Here are some tips for fortifying your strengths for future success:

> Spend time with someone who shares your mission and who encourages your growth.

> Spend social time with the coworkers and teams you enjoy being with.

> When possible, dress for the job you want, not the one you have.

> Look at your job. If you are unemployed, look at a prior job or the way you spend your time—attending school, working at home. Use that as your job.

Fitting In and Standing Out: Important Tips for Landing the Job

Getting a job has two major parts. The first part is getting past the gatekeeper. Only 20 percent of applicants get an interview. The gatekeeper's job is to keep you from getting an interview. In larger companies, gatekeeping is usually a function of the HR department. This is where your résumé is screened and initial decisions are made. In today's environment, job applications must be cut down to a manageable number for the actual hiring people to interview and make a decision. To get past the gatekeeper, you need to have the qualifications for the job and probably not wave any red flags. Here, the emphasis is on fitting in. Remember, the gatekeeper's job is to look for reasons to reject your application.

The second part of getting a job is to be the one selected out of the few individuals who get past the gatekeeper. Here it is important to stand out, to be unique, and to offer talents and skills that justify your selection for the position. People who hire you will be looking to see how you can make them look better, not at how competent you are in your own right (although people tend to think that the prospect's competence is the deciding factor). The people who make the actual hiring decisions or recommendations may not be aware of the factors that influence their choices. If you look too strong or too well-qualified or too ambitious, you may be perceived as a threat to the person who has the greatest influence on the hiring decision.

Incredibly, 80 percent of available jobs are never advertised. When networking, rather than asking a contact if he or she has any job openings, it is more effective to ask, "Do you know of any organizations that might be hiring?" Don't put a person on the spot, but do indicate that you are looking for job possibilities. Even go so far as to add, "If you hear of something that I might be interested in, please let me know. Here is my contact information (my card)." Then change the subject to something the contact is interested in.

Building a Portfolio and Your Self-Regard

Develop a portfolio by collecting everything you can remember, even if you don't have the dates. Include information about your current or most recent employer: start date, starting pay, end date, salary. Include a company description, job titles, and major duties and responsibilities. Include work samples. List skills, achievements, contributions, compliments and recognition received, organizational levels of people interacted with, and personal characteristics that facilitated your work, such as the following:

> Analytical/judgment skills
> Teamwork and chemistry with coworkers
> Communication skills
> Poise and confidence
> Dedication
> Energy, drive, and determination
> Economy and efficiency
> Integrity

- Pride and motivation
- Following protocol
- Consistency, seeing projects through
- Quality and compliance
- Reflections on successes
- Educational history
- Military experience
- Language fluency
- Computer expertise
- Publications
- Interests
- Memberships and professional associations
- Volunteer work
- Descriptions of how you have made a difference

After building a master portfolio with every imaginable fact, fashion a targeted résumé for each position you are interested in. Limit it to one page for every 10 years of experience.

Along with bolstering your confidence with an updated résumé, you can improve your energy and outlook on the job hunt by implementing the five PERMA factors. The Positivity Academy (Morgan, 2013) provides tools and activities to support the acquisition of new ways of seeing and new skills. PERMA stands for:

- **Positive emotion.** Know what gives you pleasure and makes you feel good, like tasty foods, warm baths, a favorite book or movie, snow falling, sunshine, and the like. These are the things that deliver momentary happiness and life satisfaction; they are important markers in positive emotion.

› **Engagement.** What captures you? What makes you lose track of time while you are completely absorbed in a fulfilling experience or challenging task? This is about the experience of *flow,* and it is a time when self-consciousness is lost.

› **Relationships.** Positive relationships and social ties are extremely reliable indicators of happiness. Other people are the best antidote to the downs of life and the single most reliable up.

› **Meaning.** Belonging to and serving something that you believe is bigger than yourself are essential ingredients in happiness and well-being. Meaning may be determined both subjectively and objectively. Connections to others give life meaning and purpose.

› **Accomplishments.** Realizing tangible goals and undertaking activities that we choose for their own sake, free of coercion, deliver happiness and well-being. We would do them with or without reward, because they are our calling and our passion.

For more job-search advice and tips, visit www.positivityacademy.com.

Annie's Story

I had been on Vicodin for almost 6 months because I had injured my knee. I had gone to my supervisor and said I had a problem with taking pain pills on the job. I wondered if there was any help for me. The pills were prescribed. The surgeon just kept giving me pain pills. I didn't know anything about addiction at the time. I didn't realize I was addicted. When I took Vicodin, I remember thinking, "This must be what normal people feel like." The surgeon kept prescribing them, and I kept taking them.

After about a month, I went back to my supervisor and said, "I'm taking these at work, is this okay?" She said, "Let me check on it." She called the board of nursing. They said as long as I was seeing an addictionologist or someone who specialized in addiction who knew about the prescription, it was okay. This was in about 1992.

I tried to stop, many times. I set up a tapering schedule. It didn't work. I tried to stop probably 10 times a day and could not. I decided I was going to take a month off to get well. I was willing to do whatever it took to get well—including getting sick. I was seeing a psychiatrist at the time who knew what was going on. She said she would help me. She put me on clonidine. I didn't know what withdrawal was going to be like. It was awful. The physical complaints, the restlessness, the anxiety, feeling like you're going to jump out of your skin! Everything felt so bad. I called her saying, "I can't do this." She replied, "Well tough. You have to. You have to buck up and just do it." She was almost mean to me. There was no empathy or anything.

I took it upon myself to call in a prescription to a K-Mart pharmacy, using a patient's name from the cancer center where I worked. As I walked out the door, two police officers confronted me. To this day, I don't know how, but I got out of it. I went to the home of the patient for whom I had called in the prescription and told her what I had done. I remember she said to me, "If you needed medicine, you should've just asked me. I would've given it to you."

It was horrible to think what I did to her. Of course they found out at work. That's how they caught me. The pharmacist at K-Mart called where I worked and reported that a prescription had been called in for this patient. They checked it out and discovered it was me.

I was called in to meet with the the nurse administrator, my immediate supervisor, and HR. They were pretty threatening. They told me if I didn't surrender my license, they would press charges. My immediate supervisor, the one I had gone to earlier for help, said, "Don't ever step foot on this campus again."

When I told my husband, he was shocked. He had no idea. We both decided I would turn in my license to the board. That's when I went in the first time to the recovering nurse program (PRN). Being fired was the worst experience of my life. The day I left, they changed all the locks on the doors and the pharmacy doors.

That time of my life was horrible. I was sober for only 3 months when I got pregnant. I had no nursing license. I couldn't find a job. I saw an ad in the paper and went to work for people selling meat off the back of a truck. The good news was that I had stopped using before I got pregnant. If I'd gotten pregnant before getting into PRN, I don't think I could've stopped.

After my first treatment program, I thought I was embracing recovery, but I never put it first in my life. It was maybe third or fourth on the list of priorities. I didn't take it as seriously as I should have. I just figured, "Oh I'm sober now, and that'll be fine."

I went to meetings, and I went to my first outpatient program. It was really hard then because I had a new baby, a very difficult, colicky baby, and I didn't want to leave her with anyone else. At that time, I didn't think I was using it as an excuse, but I probably was. I relapsed before I even finished my first treatment program. I relapsed on cough medicine. It had hydrocodone in it. I had dirty urine. I remember the medical director from the lab calling. I made up some elaborate story. I'm sure he was thinking, "Sure, I've heard this one before."

I was in my second treatment program. I was working in a doctor's office and would take the narcotic samples for personal use. We did pilot physicals exams. I scammed on my urines by using theirs. They were clean 99 percent of the time, until we had a dirty pilot. That's how I got caught the third time.

I remember the interventionist saying to me, "This is your third relapse. You are either going to give up your license or do something." I had no idea that "something" meant I was going to leave my child and go away for 3½ months. My sister did all the research and told me the same thing, "Whatever you're doing, it's not working, and you have to go." I fought it. "No, I'm not going. No way am I going. You can't make me go. I'm not going." But I went! For over 3 months! My sister managed to rally up enough money in a short period of time from all of my family members and my husband's family members and bought me a plane ticket.

I was still in withdrawal when I got to the recovery center. The cost was $25,000, but if you had to go to their hospital for withdrawal, it was an additional $10,000. So I detoxed at home. I remember how miserable I was. I could hardly walk. I could hardly get on the plane. I knew I couldn't use because I didn't want my family to pay another $10,000.

I didn't think this would be so hard. I haven't talked about this in such a long time. Talking about my family is what brings me to tears. That's what kept me sober and sticking with inpatient. I figured the best thing I could do to pay back my family was to go through the program and not to waver.

I kept thinking, "I gotta get out of here on time because there's no more money." In a way, that helped me take the program more seriously. I probably saw a couple dozen people come and go. They told us that if we completed the program, 85–90% would stay sober. But if we didn't, many would end up dead. It was like the last-stop place to go. That scared me!

Being away from my baby was really hard. She still to this day remembers me crying on the couch. She was only 2½ years old, and she has a very distinct memory of that time before I went to treatment. Me crying on the couch. She knew something was really wrong, and she always felt sick because I would just sit on the couch and cry. That was when I was going through withdrawal. When I came home, she asked me if I was all better or if I was going to get sick again. I told her I was all better. She said, "Let me look at your eyes." So in the past, she knew that something was wrong. She could see it in my eyes—probably that dead look you get when you're stoned.

The treatment center was a good place for me to go because recovery, for the first time in my life, was my priority. I had to go to a meeting every day. It was like being in the military. It was what I needed. I was forced to do all those things that I never did when I had a choice. The people I met there changed me too. I could see where a person could end up. I saw people who had money to burn, people who hadn't lost everything, how it kept them sick. They knew that if they didn't go through this program, they would just go to another. They hadn't lost everything. During my stay there, my house was sold. There were garage sales, selling off all my belongings. I came home to no house. The price we paid for my recovery was tremendous.

My husband and family came down for family week. My mother thought they were going to blame her for my disease. My mom and dad became really good friends with a few other couples there. One of the couples had a son, a cardiologist. It really helped my parents. They realized that addiction happens in every socioeconomic class, and these two people were wonderful parents, like mine were. It really was therapeutic for them to realize this is a problem that is everywhere. It's not just scumbag people, like my parents believed. I think it was helpful for them. My parents never drank. There was never alcohol in our home, ever. It was hard for them to wrap around the idea of a daughter as a drug addict. They're all very religious. That's their addiction.

Sometimes I still want to drink—like socially, at a party. But I don't drink because I remember the last time I thought that was okay. We were camping and it was hot. I thought, "I'll just have a beer. What's that going to hurt?" Alcohol's never been my thing. But after a couple of months, I was using again. What I know now is just do what you're told. Until I embraced recovery, I never did.

References

Morgan, D.L. (2013). *Unalienable pursuits, module 6: In pursuit of career fulfillment.* Clarion, PA: Positivity Academy.

8

for coworkers, managers, and monitors

When it comes to addressing substance use disorder (SUD) issues, some medical professionals will respond with understanding and support for treatment, while others will react from prejudice and insufficient education. It's ironic that well-educated, scientifically minded, and research-based professionals are relatively new to the recognition, education, and treatment of colleagues with SUDs. It just goes to show that it is one thing to intellectually agree with something (like the DSM V) and quite another to effect systemic behavioral changes. Fortunately, there is power in knowledge. And for those reading this book, your knowledge will help power the change toward healthier responses to colleagues who are suffering from substance use disorder.

This chapter provides information for nurse managers and colleagues of nurses with substance use disorders (SUDs). Topics include signs of impairment, addressing concerns, the legal obligation of colleagues and managers, and how to support newly recovering nurses in the workplace.

Bringing Professional Substance Abuse Out of the Shadows

Remember hiding under the blanket at night alone in your room? If you couldn't see the monsters, they couldn't see you. You were safe. Scared, but safe from detection and harm. Even as adults, it can feel that sometimes, we want to keep the covers pulled up over our heads. There are a lot of great reasons we would rather avoid looking at what's really out there. We're busy. We're already maxed out. We're overworked, understaffed, fatigued, and running on caffeine. Who has the resources to add one more thing—especially something emotionally, legally, and logistically challenging? Inevitably, when faced with a coworker who may have SUD, the rationalizing goes like this: "She is a great nurse. This is my friend. It can't be true. We've been in the trenches together for years. She's probably just in a rough patch. We all go through those. Besides, I don't know what to say if I'm not 100% sure. I'm good at caring, not confronting. This is so bad for business. I'm not really sure. There's all that paperwork and for what? If I'm wrong, I could ruin a career here...."

Why so much ambivalence? For one thing, there is little education or emphasis on addiction and SUDs. Raise your hand if you were cautioned in nursing school about SUDs as a professional liability, complete with drills, binders, hard hats, tool belts, and safety ropes. Did you leave school confident about how to safeguard yourself or discuss nurses' vulnerability to substance abuse with a colleague? Perhaps like some students, the extent of your SUD education consisted of a paragraph about drug or alcohol use in the pharmacology lecture at nursing school. And when you started your first job, did you pay more than cursory attention to the paragraphs regarding SUD in the workplace during your orientation?

NOTE | *As mentioned in Chapter 1, "The Bottom Dropped Out," imagine avoiding the topic of crash-landing a plane in flight school. The crash statistics are far below 10 percent for pilots, and yet 10 percent or more of nurses will crash due to SUDs!*

SUDs are both costly and lethal, so much so that they warrant greater attention and stronger measures from all health care fronts, including education, administration, and treatment plans. According to the National Drug Control Strategy, "Illicit drug use in America contributed to an estimated $193 billion in crime, health, and lost productivity costs in 2007, the year for which the most recent estimate is available" (National Drug Control Strategy, 2012, p. 3).

TIP | *To increase your understanding and empathy regarding nurses susceptible to SUDs, refer to the sections "Join the Club" and "The Perfect Storm: Opportunity, Means, and Motive" in Chapter 1.*

Certified Alcohol Drug Counselor (CADC) Jeanette Flood, who has worked with hundreds of nurses over her more than 40 years in drug/alcohol treatment, states: "To have more understanding of chemical dependency, nurse practicum should include a minimum of 12 AA and Al-Anon meetings. Student nurses should attend 2 meetings a week for a period of 6 weeks. At the end of the 6 weeks, they would then write a paper on the first step of

AA and something they feel powerless about!" (personal communication, 2013). Flood's recommendation is further supported in a study by Martinez and Murphy-Parker. The purpose of their study was to examine two methods of teaching nursing students about alcohol addiction. They concluded:

> Group 1 received lecture only, whereas group 2 received lecture and discussion with a person who had been sober for many years. Both groups showed improved scores in knowledge and certain aspects of beliefs; however, group 2 showed greater knowledge and more accurate beliefs overall toward this population than group 1. The introduction of a person successfully remaining sober was shown to be an even more effective teaching strategy than lecture alone (2003, p. 156).

Employers and patients don't want to view their caretakers as risky. Nurses certainly don't want to view themselves as putting patients at risk. Nurses want to see themselves as compassionate, capable, intelligent people who put patient welfare first. Combine good intentions with sparse SUD education, punitive responses to self-reporting, varying degrees of helper-profession codependent traits (refer to the section "Codependency" in Chapter 6, "Reentry and the Return Home"), employer ambivalence, cultural dysfunctions, legalities and privacy rights, and it's no wonder that, collectively, we get poor marks. Indeed, "The nurses in one particular study indicated that there was a culture of mistreatment of addicts as patients in the workplace by health care professionals. Not surprisingly, this culture or stigma was listed as a prevailing reason for the nurses' own concealment of their problem from their colleagues" (NCSBN, 2011, p. 49).

Bringing the topic of nurses with SUDs out of the shadows and into the forefront of education and management will save lives, increase patient safety, and position nurses to lead society in better addressing addiction and SUD. Becoming more skilled at addressing SUD with compassion, clarity, and boundaries can help develop managerial competence. If you are already a skilled communicator with healthy boundaries, you will be more adept at training your staff to address SUD issues more effectively. We discuss leadership practices in more depth later in this chapter and in Chapter 9, "Leadership and a Culture for Recovery," much of which was contributed by Dr. Cynthia Clark.

For the most part, society has counted on local, state, and federal governments to deal with substance abuse problems. Lawmakers are beginning to respond to the crisis with a new type of state legislation relating to how painkillers are prescribed, largely in response to the increasing epidemic of misuse and over prescription of painkillers—and the commensurate costs in overdoses and pill mills (Grill, 2013). Grill says that "nationwide, more than 116 million Americans struggle with chronic pain each year. In 2008, painkillers were linked to 14,800 overdose deaths—more than for heroin and cocaine combined—and more than 12 million people reported using prescription painkillers for unintended reasons in 2010" (¶ 2). Further, Grill reports that the quantity of prescription painkillers sold to pharmacies, hospitals, and physicians' offices quadrupled from 1999 to 2010. "In fact, the supply that year [2010] was enough to medicate every American adult for one month with painkillers" (¶ 2).

Aside from legislative action, more is needed. It is time for health care professionals to face these problems within our own ranks and take action. We can't wait any longer for effective solutions to deal with prevention, reclamation of people suffering from SUDs, and early sobriety support. As we have emphasized throughout this book, prescription drug overdosing is now the leading cause of accidental death in the United States. That should get our attention. We're not talking about drug lords killing us with street drugs. If you were leading a task force to investigate the contributing factors that make prescription drugs the leading cause of accidental death, what would you want to know? Here are a few questions:

> How many people died taking drugs that were prescribed to them?
> Conversely, how many people died taking drugs that were not prescribed to them? Where did they get them?
> Why do so many people accidentally take fatal dosages?
> Why do we have such an alarming rate of deaths from medications that are meant to help us?
> What is our responsibility to the public we serve?
> Are we responsibly prescribing medication?
> What will prevent and reduce the rate of accidental prescription drug overdoses?

If there was news of a growing plague that was killing millions and costing billions, wouldn't lawmakers, law enforcers, and medical professionals marshal forces to counter the epidemic? Not only do we need to become professionally more proactive for the public's sake, we need to do better by our own colleagues who are afflicted. Godfrey et al (2010, p. 2) found that "[s]tates with disciplinary programs that focused on deterrence and punishment prohibited employment of these nurses, which resulted in the loss of the nurses' health insurance and financial means to recover. Alternative programs treat impaired nurses as individuals who have a treatable, chronic disease. Policymakers in states with alternative therapy programs believe in a more humane, rehabilitative approach for nurses with substance use disorders."

When we interviewed nurses for this book, a number of them voiced the following sentiment: Why can nurses care for patients, but when they become patients (with SUDs), nurses are uncared for? It is easy to see the irony in this situation and imagine the pain of feeling more tainted by stigma than supported by your peers. Let's follow that irony by a second—

nurses with SUDs don't always treat themselves well, but they want their colleagues to treat them well. Poor self-care and dubious boundary setting are two common culprits contributing to substance abuse. It's a tough spot to be in. The good news in all of this leads us to the greatest irony of all: Poor self-care and having an SUD can ultimately lead to a healthier life. If any person with addiction issues wants a life of recovery, that life calls for constant and never-ending improvement. Let's put it another way: If I'm afflicted with substance use disorder and I want to achieve well-being, I am coerced into taking care of myself. Let's review: *Health* care professionals are learning to be healthier.

Roles and Responsibilities for Managers and Coworkers

Regardless of whether you are working with nurses in recovery, it is generally good business to increase your awareness and observation skills concerning the demeanor, disposition, and performance of your colleagues. This applies to earlier detection of substance abuse, acknowledging a job well done, and monitoring a nurse in the early recovery. Here is a handy acronym from international intervention specialist John Southworth, who notes that "Being an old sheepherder, I came up with BAAA as a way to remember [the following]":

> Behaviors
> Attitude
> Achievement
> Attendance

For each nurse on your team, note a baseline for his or her BAAA attributes, as well as any changes in their norms. That is a great way to home in on potential reasons for concern and greater discernment. It is also a way to recognize and acknowledge noteworthy performance. For more specific guidance in dealing with substance abuse issues, note your primary resources, which we call the Four Principals:

> The Nurse Practice Act (for your state)
> *SUD Manual Guidelines* from NCSBN (NCSBN Primary Directive)
> BON website
> Your agency's policies and procedures

Within the boundaries of these four principal resources, you can address substance abuse in a responsive manner or a reactionary one. These two approaches are distinguished by the level of informal or formal action required. The first approach is using a check-in to address or respond to questionable provocations. In the second approach, you are required to react to evidence of substance abuse with a confrontation or an intervention.

NOTE

The National Council for State Boards of Nursing (NCSBN) came out of the American Nurses Association (ANA). The ANA is the voice and lobby of nursing in Washington, D.C. According to its website, the primary goal of NCSBN is to protect the public and to ensure public safety.

Responsive Behavior: The Check-In

Responsive behavior is characterized by the check-in. For a check-in, you must be paying attention to your colleague's overall mental state, as well as any attitude or behavior shifts. Being aware of changes enables you to respond to your coworker. Do this by checking in to see if anything is wrong. This check-in is comparable to looking in on a patient whose vital signs have changed. While there might not be any real threat, you want to monitor changes to make sure your patient is tended to and that things do not adversely progress without your awareness, as that could limit treatment options later. You also want your patient to take appropriate action in his or her own interests—for example, getting proper rest, getting hydrated, eating properly, attending physical therapy, and the like. The idea is to hold up a mirror that reflects concern, curiosity, and clarity:

> **Concern for a colleague/friend:** "I want good things for you."

> **Curiosity about what you're seeing:** "Something's different. What am I seeing, hearing, sensing?"

> **Clarity:** "I see you. Your behaviors are noticeable," or "We have inherent risks and responsibilities in nursing," or "We can help each other."

Check-ins are opportunities for colleagues to reinforce a culture of support and awareness, which can help deter a nurse from sliding from substance abuse to addiction.

At this stage, there are no work-site infractions that require action. The check-in might go like this:

> I've noticed lately that you don't quite seem like yourself. You seem out of character, and I'm a little concerned. I've worked with you for 3 years and respect you and your nursing. I've never known you to be so forgetful or reactionary as you have been lately. Hearing you be short with coworkers and patients caught my attention. On top of that, I've heard you repeating the same question the past couple of days. For some of our staff, this might sound normal. For you it is really different. This behavior just isn't like you. Last time I observed these kinds of changes it was due to substance abuse. As difficult as this is for me to bring up, I can't look the other way if you are in trouble. Do you need any help or support?

VOICES

It's always good to lead with your emotions. Nobody can argue with your emotions. Now, they may argue with what you're interpreting, but they can't argue with, "I'm worried about you. I'm concerned." So, "I'm worried" can begin a conversation and keep the door open."

–Mark H. Broadhead, MD

Reactionary Behavior: Reacting to Signs of Substance Abuse

In this scenario, you react to signs of substance abuse through intervention or confrontation. You can try to intervene on—or call a stop to—poor performance that may result from substance abuse outside of work. In this case, you are giving a nurse a warning (formal or informal). For example, perhaps you smell alcohol on a nurse, he has repeatedly come in to work appearing hungover, and he has increasing absenteeism. If the behavior continues or escalates, your attempt to intervene and stop the behavior now evolves into a confrontation. This is a formal meeting, including agency staff (such as HR or the director of nursing) to confront the nurse in question with evidence of using, diverting, or being impaired while on the job. At this point, you are part of a formal process to address the issue and take proper steps to ensure public safety.

To review the stages in addressing substance abuse:

> In the early stages, you address a shift in behavior, attitude, achievement, or attendance to check in with a nurse. Using BAAA markers, you have a good reference point to use as your baseline.

> If indicators are more pronounced, you intervene by calling out the issues and discuss future consequences.

> If behaviors have escalated into legal, ethical, or workplace violations, you now confront the nurse with evidence, and consequences become real.

Reporting Guidelines

In an ideal world, early detection would be the emphasis. You could spot and address precursory tendencies before they grew into full-fledged addictions. Until that ideal world exists, here are some universal guidelines for reporting suspicions of on-the-job impairment:

> Know the Nurse Practice Act. Be aware of what it says about a nurse's duty to report unethical behavior, unprofessional behavior, or conduct that appears to be a result of substance abuse. There may be a legal duty to report, as patient protection is paramount. Failure to report could result in discipline or sanction from the board of nursing. If ethics aren't inducement enough, there could be legal liability for the institution as well as the nurse. If patient safety and ethics aren't inducement enough to report prohibited behavior, protect yourself. You could potentially lose your job, lose your license, and face imprisonment. Who wants to experience years of regret about not saying something earlier?

> Follow your institution's reporting policies and procedures.

> Report to the designated staff member, such as the nurse manager or chief nursing officer.

> Keep discussions confidential. This is not a matter for gossip or something to process with a colleague. If you start telling other people things you're not sure about, it could lead to legal liability such as defamation. There is no off-hand version of "Do you think Mary is using? Because I think she might be." Mary could be experiencing side effects of some legitimate medication that mimics substance abuse, such as fatigue (nodding off), imbalance, or slurred speech.

> Articulate in clear, specific terms "enough" of any of the following: facts, observations of behaviors (unusual, inconsistent conduct), or physical evidence.

Potential Signs of Substance Abuse

Being able to describe what you're seeing is important for checking in and addressing concerns. As a nurse, you are adept at describing symptoms. Included here is a list of common attributes that can indicate substance abuse. Coworkers and supervisors must be able to identify the various ways chemical dependence can manifest in the nurse. Any of the following can occur, alone or in combination (Angres, Bettinardi-Angres, & Talbott, 1998):

> Cognitive impairment
> Excessive tardiness or absenteeism
> Mood swings
> Appearance changes
> Increase in personal problems, such as financial difficulty or divorce
> Increase in physical complaints
> Dilated or pinpoint pupils
> Excessive weight loss or gain
> Needle marks
> Wearing long sleeves all the time to avoid needle-mark detection
> Spending excessive time around opioids
> Working too many hours (perhaps for greater access to opioids to avoid withdrawal symptoms)
> Asking physicians for prescriptions
> Colleagues noting opioids missing in the workplace

Other signs include the following:

> Slurred speech
> Memory problems
> Dizziness
> Depression
> Sedation/drowsiness
> Confusion
> Constipation
> Slowed breathing
> Lack of coordination
> Reduced sense of pain

As noted by Talbert (2009):

> Many signs and symptoms of substance abuse are general, non-specific, and easily hidden. However, over time, an individual's behavior paints a clearer picture. "Nurses with substance dependency often use before and during their shifts" (Ponech, 2000, p. 17). Additional indicators include...excessive amounts of time spent in medication rooms or near medication carts, work performance that alternates between high and low productivity, and inattention or poor judgment (Drug Enforcement Administration [DEA], 2008). Other signs of substance abuse include damaged relationships among colleagues, friends, and patients; heavy "wastage" of drugs...and increased concerns voiced by patients.

Common signs of an impending relapse include the following (National Council of State Boards of Nursing, 2011):

> Lack of a sober support system and a return to socializing with prior using associates
> Decreased participation in an ongoing recovery program, including a 12-step program, and a lack of a sponsor relationship
> Failing to comply with treatment recommendations
> Failing to comply with alternative-to-discipline contract requirements
> Lack of honesty regarding substance use and misuse history
> Employment difficulties
> Relationship difficulties
> Unstable emotional status
> Late or missing monitoring reports
> Missed drug screens
> Diluted specimens
> Altered or substituted specimens
> Positive drug screens

173

Hiring

Why hire a nurse with substance use disorder? If you are skeptical, first consider whether you would want to be eligible for hire if *you* were afflicted with SUD. No one is immune. There are nurses who never drank or used in their lives who developed the disease by taking prescribed medication. At some point, the dosage increased to match the increase in tolerance as the patient slid into danger during the course of neurological synaptic downregulation.

Downregulation

The process of downregulation is a major contributor to becoming addicted to a substance. The phenomenon of downregulation is described by Hanson (2011) as the following:

> When we take drugs continuously, the brain compensates for the artificial flood of, or sensitivity to, serotonin, dopamine, and other neurotransmitters by cutting back on its own production, and the receptors on the cell surfaces ultimately degrade...The concern with downregulation is that, over time, chronic use of serotonin reuptake blockers or dopamine-active drugs of abuse can lead to both a decrease in the number of receptors and a desensitization of existing receptors.

The brain does not stay idle during these artificial rains of neurotransmitters. As explained by Peter Kramer in *Listening to Prozac*, "The chronic, constant, reliable presence of high levels of neurotransmitter causes the cell to downregulate." In layman's terms, the patient needs higher doses to experience less effect. Downregulation is a significant ingredient in addiction.

In the midst of our national substance abuse epidemic, it may be interesting to know that patients and coworkers may be safer working with nurses who are being monitored. That is largely because the increase in underreported substance abuse is becoming a significant concern. "Workplace interventions for substance use and abuse have been in place through employee assistance programs (EAPs) for some time, but these resources are historically underutilized and most workers remain unidentified and underreported, particularly nurses" (National Council of State Boards of Nursing,

2011, p. 51). Furthermore, "when employers have pro-active policies and procedures in place that acknowledge the existence of these disorders in the nursing work force, identification and referral is enhanced, leading to safer work conditions and improved employee morale" (Indiana State Nurses Assistance Program for Nurses, 2011, ¶3).

Reasons to Hire a Recovering Nurse

From the Indiana State Nurses Assistance Program (ISNAP) for Nurses:

> When employers retain or hire an ISNAP nurse, they have a nurse with an identified risk who is closely monitored, including random drug testing and a work-site monitor. The nurse applicant who is less known, i.e., not in ISNAP, may seem more desirable but may actually prove to have more liabilities. Research has shown that nurses in alternative programs (vs. nurses under licensure discipline) not only return to practice sooner but also if relapse occurs, they are identified sooner providing less risk of harm. The caveat for employers: Be Careful! Being more punitive and restrictive may cause you to go from the frying pan to the fire! (Indiana State Nurses Assistance Program for Nurses, 2011, ¶6).

VOICES

> I've worked in a number of places—general medical settings, psychiatric settings, and general psychiatry settings—where we have had recovering nurses (and the ones we've had have been excellent to work with). Part of working with patients involves being able to sit in the same room with someone who's in pain. If you've never been in pain or worked through your own pain, it's very difficult to sit in a room and just be with them. Although that's not the end-all, be-all of psychiatric work, it's kind of a prerequisite and a necessity to be able to do good work. Again, it goes back to the whole idea between sympathy and empathy. I can have empathy for your pain, and yet I also have the emotional reserve and ability to do the next right thing in terms of therapy.
>
> –Mark H. Broadhead, MD

Medical professionals interviewed for this book (personal communication, 2013) volunteered an additional reason they hire nurses in recovery. To summarize: People in recovery are required to undergo an extensive treatment program centered on personal growth and high levels of personal accountability. Many people who stay in recovery model exemplary behavior and become role models on the job and in their social communities.

Hiring nurses in recovery can be an excellent choice. And as with any potential candidate, it is invaluable to use careful consideration and screening during the hiring process. If interviewees disclose that they are currently under contract with the state board and participating in a recovery program, know the legal boundaries. If you haven't already, confirm with HR what topics and questions are legally acceptable to ask regarding their BON contract and any license restrictions. (To see a list of self/work appraisal questions for nurses in recovery who are pursuing employment, see the section "Questions to Ask Yourself" in Chapter 7, "Careers and Change."

We caution you to pay attention to the applicant who seems extraordinarily confident and portrays immunity to old traps and triggers. It is a good sign if he or she anticipates risks and has thought out ways to mitigate them. Take, for instance, the example of a recovering alcoholic. Most of the millions of recovering alcoholics have not given up shopping in a grocery store because there's a beer and wine section. What they have done is anticipated the hotspots and entered with a strong strategy to avoid being seduced into relapse. Hence, we have millions who can successfully navigate the grocery store without relapsing after every shopping trip. Likewise, a potential employee with a good recovery program will anticipate the old trigger zones (the Pyxis machine, sample packets, ampules breaking open, the smell of an alcohol swab) and plan how to mitigate any relapse risk. If a candidate hasn't thought through workplace risks and the recovery strategies, he or she might be more preoccupied with getting hired than maintaining recovery.

VOICES

A positive sign that someone is doing well is that he is open about his disease. He is forthcoming with details, if you wish. By the same token, he is not wearing it on his sleeve. This tends to indicate that he is comfortable with the fact that he has a disease and is comfortable enough to be responsible about it with strangers, bosses, and managers. He's somebody who has a sense of place with it. What I mean by that is that he's not running back to work simply because he needs the money. There's a sense of gratitude in the fact that, "I get to do this." Not, "I have to do this."

There are two sides to this. One can be overly grateful for it and thus be a doormat. "Sure, I'll take whatever shift you've got, whatever time you've got—anything. I'll take anything!" That doesn't mean you don't take them, but it does mean they've got some work to do and you've got to watch them. These are the people who are apt to burn out quickly, too. They will take anything, they will do anything, and that's often what got them in trouble to begin with. So they're not able to care for themselves.

You want somebody who is glad they have a job, who's grateful, and yet is also able to say, "No, that's not good for me." This is a sense of place and a sense of balance.

–Mark H. Broadhead, MD

Work-Site Monitoring

There are two distinct types of monitoring for nurses with SUDs. Most of the monitoring mentioned throughout this book refers to the monitor assigned by the state board to oversee your contract. This monitor may be an employee or contractor of the state board. The second tier of monitoring can be overseen by a designated supervisor at your workplace, often referred to as a work-site monitor. The majority of nurses who enroll in an alternative-to-discipline program are required to have their work monitored by a supervisor—often, and preferably, a nurse. "Worksite monitors are in a position to assist recovering nurses to remain in the workforce and to ensure patient safety through a program of close monitoring" (Young, 2008). They understand the disease of addiction, can recognize the signs of SUD, and can respond appropriately.

> Organized education for professionals who serve as worksite monitors is important in order to ensure consistent reporting to boards and for effective monitoring of impaired nurses who return to practice. Successful development and implementation of these programs benefit patient safety, nurses, worksite monitors and boards of nursing (Young, 2008).

A work-site monitor will obviously require clear written guidelines to fulfill the legal and professional expectations of this role. We also recommend being knowledgeable of, and following guidelines from, the Four Principals. (As mentioned earlier in this chapter, these principals are the Nurse Practice Act for your state, *SUD Manual Guidelines* from NCSBN, the BON website for your state, and your agency's policies and procedures.)

If you agree to be a work-site monitor, aside from monitoring a nurse's work performance and tracking signs of responsible recovery in the workplace, there is a rich opportunity to be a resource for encouragement and development to the nurse in recovery.

TIP | *If you find yourself assigned to be a work-site monitor, refer to the sections "Reporting Guidelines" and "Potential Signs of Substance Abuse" earlier in this chapter for helpful information. In addition, you'll find relapse indicators on page 141 of the SUD Manual Guidelines from NCSBN, as well as in this chapter's section "Potential Signs of Substance Abuse."*

VOICES

One thing I think is important for a monitor to be able to do is catch the nurse doing something good. "You seem to be having a good day today. How is that?" If they're used to those types of conversations, it's also easier to say, "You seem to be having a bad day today. What's going on?" So it's more of an ongoing conversation than it is the grand inquisition about the current emotional state. It's okay to hang out in the principal's office when the principal asks you, "You seem to be doing good. What's going on? How is that?" If you can share in their joy, they'll share their pain with you as well.

One of the things I think is important not only for nurses to know but also for nurse managers is that those of us with addictions—especially in the medical field—are very type A. We're very good at what we've done. We want to read the book, take the test, get the A, and move on. And that's what we think: "At the end of this procedure, we will have a well patient, and then we're done," as opposed to the idea of looking at it as more of a chronic disease, like the diabetic who's always going to have to take the insulin. Unlike diabetes, however, the longer you treat this disorder, the better you can get. But that takes time. We often beat ourselves up because we're not perfect yet, and we can project that out. Our monitors can pick up on that and conclude, "They're not well yet. This doesn't look like it's working." The more appropriate perspective is to view the nurse as someone recuperating from trauma. Some days are going to be better than others.

That's a problem sometimes for people who are monitoring or people who are hiring. "How well do they have to be before we can hire them? I want them well first." No, you want them well enough.

–Mark H. Broadhead, MD

Confronting a Nurse with Substance Use Infractions

It can be alarming to be called by the CNO into a confrontation with a staff member, "stat." But with an estimated 10% of nurses suffering from SUDs, there are good odds of participating in such an event. If you are unprepared, you will be grasping for a hold on your role. If, however, you are prepared, you will be effective as a leader and an advocate for your nurse, your institution, and the profession. You will better understand your role and how to help a nurse who is in trouble, whether the trouble is substance abuse or an incorrect accusation. Either way, you can best serve the process by being prepared and, therefore, having your staff prepared.

TIP

Does your agency have a substance abuse committee? If not, research ways to get this instituted. We strongly urge you to include a nurse advocate and someone with recovery experience on the committee. A nurse advocate can make recommendations to the committee, offer guidance for interventions, and be a resource for a confronted nurse. Possible roles for an SUD committee include reviewing cases for intervention and action, providing educational support for managers, and coordinating an outreach program with local nurse educators on the topic of SUD. For a list of potential roles for an SUD committee, see page 65 of the NCSBN SUD Manual Guidelines in the section on SUD intervention committees.

One tool to assist a manager and nurse during a confrontation is to have a binder prepared. The binder would include the following three sections.

- > Our Agency
- > Manager Information
- > Staff Packet

Section 1: Our Agency

This section in your binder is a placeholder for institutional information such as your company's vision, mission, and core principles, along with the rules of engagement, policies, and procedures. The purpose is to always have on hand the cultural umbrella under which you are working. You can refer to the agency's vision, mission, and core values to check that the leadership decisions you make and the actions you take are properly aligned. It is good to begin a conversation with, "According to the mission to 'empower employees to professional excellence,' it is important that I not ignore when one of you is struggling. Today, I want to talk to you about... ."

Section 2: For Managers

This section in your binder lists useful information you need to fulfill your role and outlines your plan to educate your staff and establish a restorative culture for nurses. It should include the following:

> A copy of the Nurse Practice Act

> State board of nursing approach (is yours a discipline or alternative state). Refer to Chapter 3, "Getting Back to Work," to review the information on state-based SUD recovery approaches.

> Questions to ask the employer's agent (nurse manager or CNO and HR) prior to confrontation. These might include the following:

>> "Can you please clarify your expectations of my role during the confrontation?"

>> "What is required of me by our institution and the board of nursing?"

>> "Is there a nurse advocate who is available to the nurse after the confrontation?"

> Phone numbers for an intervention specialist and local peer support group facilitators

> An education calendar (When are your in-service trainings on SUD?)

> Educational materials (sample topics, role-plays, quizzes, workshops) regarding the following:

>> Agency education

>> The DESC Model for Assertive Communication; see Chapter 9, "Leadership and a Culture for Civility"

>> Prevention (early warning signs and checking in)

>> Intervention (what might happen during or after a confrontation)

> Legal ramifications and recommendations from your HR department

> NCSBN SUD Manual at https://www.ncsbn.org/SUDN_10.pdf

> Local SUD educational opportunities (university, recovery centers, interventionists)

Section 3: Staff Packet

This is a packet in your binder prepared for a nurse who is being confronted with evidence of his or her substance abuse. This packet will help you explain the process to your staff member. With the approval of HR, it should also include appropriate support options for when he or she leaves the building. The nurse could be at risk of complications from withdrawal or even suicide. (Again, before adding any of the following content to a packet, always check with HR for approval.) Content that may be helpful to a nurse with SUD can include the following:

> A list of rights

> A list of advocacy agencies

> A local peer support facilitator information packet

> A list of 12-step meetings (AA and NA)

> Phone numbers, website, and email addresses for the EAP, crisis hotlines, detox facilities, 12-step central office, a nurse advocate who's in recovery, and the state BON

> After confronting the nurse with evidence of infractions, outline the ensuing process. For example:

   1. Upon leaving this office, we will escort you to employee health for a toxicology screen.

   2. You are currently suspended from this job pending investigation.

   3. HR will provide you a cab ride home, or you can call someone to take you home.

   4. We encourage you to consider consulting the following resources when you leave here: an attorney, the state BON, the EAP, a peer-support facilitator, and a nurse in recovery. The numbers for the BON, the EAP, and HR are included in this packet.

   5. If you have drugs in your system, consider making an appointment at a detox center within the next X hours.

Best Practices and Communication

As a manager, your job is to oversee staff performance and manage the agency's expectations. As a leader, you also have the opportunity to articulate and lead from strength-based principles.

If you are interested in evolving healthier work environments, you already recognize the importance of communication. Communication is our greatest tool and our greatest challenge. Some nurses have codependent tendencies that compel them to act nice, be polite, and avoid problems that they don't know how to address. It doesn't mean there isn't a desire to improve. Often, people just don't know what to do. Many have expressed that they are uncomfortable with confrontation. How many people do you know who can tell it like it is, with clarity and without apology—just clean conversation?

A lot of times, issues aren't acknowledged because people don't know how to deal with them. For example, how many people have "the family drunk" who passes out after some obnoxious display at a reunion? Why doesn't anyone do anything to help old Uncle George? Is it because they don't love him? Is it because they don't care? Is it because they don't realize there's a problem? Most of the time, people avoid seeing what they don't feel equipped to handle.

The more you can empower your staff with strong communication tools, the more prepared they will be to address problems rather than avoiding them. The advantage is that nurses are trained observers and skilled at documentation. The challenge is that many have strong codependent traits.

The best thing you can do is build your own skills. Then, as you model desirable behaviors and walk your talk, you will shift your team culture. This is leading. Old leadership models were based on commanding from a vantage point. Today, we lead by example. "Do as I say, not as I do" never held credibility. Now that type of entitled leadership is an affront to intelligent employees.

The more you model and educate strong communication skills, the more you will establish a supportive work setting where issues are processed and morale is improved. This principle applies to all workplace issues, including substance abuse. Developing the following skills applies to all leadership concerns in addition to addressing substance abuse:

> Observe rather than interpret, judge, and gossip.

> State clean feedback versus projection and analysis. This shifts negative confrontations into conversations.

> Create a solution, plan of action, and course of treatment, including the following:

> > Clear action items

> > Clear due dates

> > Written confirmation of completion

> > Results and consequences (what is to be gained, what is to be lost)

For more leadership tools and information on creating a culture of civility, see Chapter 9.

Because this chapter is for coworkers, managers, and monitors of nurses who have issues with substance abuse, we have included both a coworker and a manager story. While most of the emotional focus of this book deals with the nurse who has SUD, it is important to recognize the emotional toll for colleagues as well. In the first story, a coworker of a nurse with SUD discusses how she felt when the problem was revealed. In the second story, a manager recounts her experiences dealing with nurses and SUDs.

Cathy, a Coworker's Story

Hindsight's 20/20. The day it happened, my friend was fired! We'd been friends for 10 years. In the last 8 months or so, I had felt myself pulling away from her because some of her choices had seemed out of character. I didn't agree with them but thought, "Well, it's not my business. I'll just step back. Not everyone does the same thing I want." She had been dating someone I didn't think was right, that kind of stuff. I told our other friend, "I'm really worried about her. She's kind of getting lost." And our friend said, "Yeah, I'm worried too. She's got one of those personalities—addictive personalities."

But when my manager told me that my friend had tried to pin her crime on me, I cried. I felt the same way as the day I found out my ex had cheated on me. I felt betrayed. They told me that she threw me under the bus. They pulled her in the office. My manager is quiet-spoken, nonthreatening. The interventionist and my manager pulled her in and approached her with, "There's been a narcotic discrepancy. Cathy's password's been used, but we have you on camera." She denied everything. She said that it was common knowledge that I gave her my password to use at any time. That it's common knowledge I give everyone my password.

Now, why I would give anyone my password? Like, here's my Social Security number, go ahead, steal my identity! Especially in our line of work. That hurt. I knew her personality. I figured it would be normal to defend yourself when caught off guard, like when you're caught speeding. That part I got. But I guess I wasn't surprised. While traveling together, I had seen her wash her Ambien down with alcohol a couple of times. I tried to approach her about it. I never thought it would cross over to that level.

Even though I understood this disease, I was tearful and questioning everything. I was shocked...but not really. She had always confided in me during difficult times in her life. After as many years as we had been friends, why couldn't she tell me? I didn't know what I was going to do. Approach her? I didn't know how.

That day, she tried to use the password again but realized it was changed. I thought, "She even tried to use it then!" And then one day when I left, she wished me a good time on my vacation. That week was her birthday. I texted her "Happy birthday!" and she wrote back, "Thanks, friend." All along she knew she was betraying me. That part hurt.

It's almost like if someone commits suicide; it's the people they leave behind who pay the price. But I keep thinking it must be a lonely place for her to be, looking over her shoulder wondering where I'm going to show up, because I'm the one person she has to face.

Margo, a Manager's Story

I never had any formal introduction in dealing with substance use, although I've been a manager for 10 years. During that time, there has been staff that I've had to discipline or let go for diversion. Early on, it was scary. It would have been helpful to know what to look for and to be able to walk through the intervention process with an experienced person.

In my first experience with substance abuse, I had to investigate an employee for possible diversion. The employee's denial was so embedded that he quit and moved to another city rather than admit to using. I learned right then that the hardest part was not being able to say anything to my staff. That put me in a difficult position.

That lesson taught me that instead of not saying anything, I can tell the staff I can't say anything. That is something I would pass on to other managers. You can share your process and reassure staff that things are getting handled. I didn't even know to say that. There have been several other cases since that time that I have told the staff, "This is being handled. I can't tell you anything because it's confidential, and if you were in this position, you would want it to be confidential." So just explaining that to the staff has been very helpful.

I'm thinking about one case in particular when I had to keep a popular nurse's diversion from the staff. This nurse was just stellar. She would help everybody, do everything. She would stay over past her shift. The staff did not believe it when they heard about her problem. That was especially true when the nurse denied what had happened and said, "No, it's not me. I didn't do that. It's the hospital framing me." That made it particularly difficult not to address the issue. After the intervention, I couldn't reveal that that nurse was sent through the program (PRN). However, she eventually came back and talked to the staff, and she now has her job back. That really gave people hope. She admitted, "I was trying to do it all."

An important but frustrating issue in an intervention is how many times I have to repeat the same thing—maybe I give it a little tweak, but it's the same thing over and over. That happened with one of the nurses who was giving fentanyl. Typically, a nurse gives half a dose at a time. Instead of hanging on to it, she should waste it. That particular nurse was keeping it. I said to the employee, "So you gave fentanyl to that patient." We'd just go over and over that scenario. I'd ask her, "What did you do with the waste? Did you waste it?" She'd say, "Yes, I did." Then I'd give another example. "Did you waste it that time?" Just the same, same, same. After about 10 times going through scenarios, she finally said, "I really didn't waste it. I didn't. I took it." I was able to say, "You have help; you can really get help." Then I reinforced how common this is and that she was not alone.

In another case, I had to confront an employee. He completely denied any using. I walked him to occupational health for a UA. There was no conversation; he didn't want to talk about anything. I tried to keep it just about process. "This is part of the process; this is what happens for anybody who we have to investigate, and this is how we do things." I think he was in a bit of shock. When we got there, he asked, "What are we doing over here again?" And I said, "Do you want me to go through it again? It's just part of the process." When he did the urine test, someone had to go in there with him, and that made him very upset. I said, "Just remember, this is part of the process. This is just how it's done. It's not personal; this is just how we do it." That reassurance was important. It was astounding to me how many times I had to tell him about the process, because he really wasn't listening. I suppose at that time, the employee is thinking ahead, "Can I get out of this, can I change the story? What can I do to save myself?"

When I asked him whom to call for a ride because his car had to stay in the parking garage, he did not want to call his wife. He did not have anybody he wanted to call. We ended up getting him a taxi home. That was a hard one. It was astounding to me how many times I had to tell him about the process.

As a manager, I notice that some in the medical field don't quite get that abuse is a disease, and that denial will kick in as part of that disease. I talked to a recovering nurse. She said that as she sat there with her manager, she was just so afraid—afraid that she would lose her whole income, that her ex-husband would take her kids. So she just shut down. She said that although she really wanted to come clean, she just felt like she couldn't.

It's not always easy to spot the red flags. I ask myself, "Is this an overachiever or a case of abuse?" I had a nurse who worked part time for years. For years, she consistently dispensed the highest percentage of narcotics on the unit. I thought, she works with high-acuity patients and all the busy hours when patients require more meds. So it was justified. But then it got so that her use increased. We saw that with the Pyxis reports. There were some behavior changes. The staff would say, " I don't know what's going on. She was really confused when I got her report." I was thinking, "Wow. Confused? That's very interesting."

I noticed that she always took her lunch at a particular time, and that was not a behavior that I had seen before. Her lunch was at about 8 p.m. The charge nurses would say, "The floor was really busy, and she took lunch then anyway." I thought, "Oh, hmm. Why?" And that was one of the things that we talked about when we confronted her—the need to take lunch at this time regardless of what was going on on the floor. That's not usual team style. She finally admitted that she had taken the drugs.

A manager needs time to prepare before engaging with the employee. I recall one incident when I was standing in the hallway with a nurse. Pharmacy called with information about some medications that were missing. The pharmacist launched into detail about a specific nurse, and she was the one with me at the time. The reporting person needs to make sure the manager is alone or has access to call the person back. Either that or the manager needs to cut the caller off and ask to call him right back. However, because you're always busy as a manager, you need to stress to a reporter that she should ask, "Is this a good time?" That would be helpful.

Each intervention has been different. But as mentioned, it's important to have a plan. Before starting the intervention, you should arrange for everyone involved to do what they need to do. We plan for HR, occupational health, and the manager(s) to be ready. We arrange to get the urinalysis done and have copies of records or charting ready. At the last intervention, I let the charge nurse know just an hour ahead: "At such and such a time, I need to talk to Jane. Have her assignment covered by so and so. This needs to be kept quiet. We want it to be seamless, and we need your help with that." I told the charge nurse there was not going to be time for the patient report and said, "You're going to have to give a report the best you can." Otherwise, the nurse would be given too much time to reconstruct her story.

One of the first things a manager can do when a nurse is being questioned is to assure him that his patients are being cared for. That puts the nurse more at ease. Also, his pager and phone should be taken away, so he knows that someone else is covering for him.

After a nurse has been enrolled in a monitoring program like the PRN, I think it's a great time to bring him back to his position or something similar because he is in counseling and having UAs. When that nurse returns, he needs a work-site monitor. It should be someone at his level or above. It should be someone who sees him frequently, so the monitor will know if he has been coming to work late or taking frequent breaks—the red flags.

Generally, returning nurses have initial restrictions such as no overtime, no weekends, no hospice, and no intensive care. But once they have some recovery under their belt, they can ask for each of those restrictions to be removed as long as they're working a good program, going to all their meetings, seeing their counselors, and attending the nurse support groups. At that point, they might say, "Can I have my weekend restrictions lifted?" Most of them don't ask for those because they think, "Hey, I don't have to work weekends for a while." Some will ask for their narcotic restriction to be lifted. When a nurse has had her restriction lifted, her manager is thinking she's actually the safest nurse we have right now, because she's in counseling and having random UAs.

Another issue for a manager to watch for is stress. Emotionally, it can be hard on the manager, because she often sees her employees as part of her family. Stress in the department should also be considered. At times we get so busy that nurses get a lot of overtime. I remember one nurse whom I worried about. It was not necessarily that she was addicted, but the potential was certainly there. I limited her, saying, "You can't work any overtime." She did not like that one bit. She would get really crabby. I said, "You're not fun to be around when you've worked extra shifts. You need to find other outlets."

Substance use disorder might have been touched on in a class, but I had no idea how much access there would be to narcotics. I wish schools would teach more about SUDs along with healthy coping skills. They don't teach coping skills. After our last episode of substance abuse, two of my new grads were talking about substance use in nursing. They said they had no idea how much risk there was.

The education or discussion of SUD is minimal, even once we're here at the hospital. I would like to see more education, whether it's an in-service or a lecture. A poster board of behaviors—even something little like that, with the EAP number on the bottom—would help, The poster could ask questions like, "Do you ever feel like this? What do you do to cope? Here are some other ideas for coping." I used to think posters were like, "Ugh, another poster." But they're bite-size pieces of information.

References

Angres, D., Bettinardi-Angres, K., and Cross, W. (1998). Nurses with chemical dependency: Promoting successful treatment and reentry. *Journal of Nursing Regulation, 1*(1),16–20.

American Psychiatric Association. (2013). *Diagnostic and Statistical Manual of Mental Disorders, 5th Edition.* Washington, DC: American Psychiatric Association

Clark, C. (2013). *Creating and Sustaining Civility in Nursing Education.* Indianapolis, IN: Sigma Theta Tau International.

Darbro N. (2005). Alternative diversion programs for nurses with impaired practice: Completers and non-completers. *Journal of Addictions Nursing, 16*(4), 169–182.

Godfrey, G., Harmon, T., Roberts, A, Spurgeon, H, McNelis, A. M., Horton-Deutsch, S. & O'Haver Day, P. (2010). Substance use among nurses. Indiana Nurses Bulletin. Retrieved from http://indiananurses.org/isnapsite/documents/2010GodfreyetalfinalcopyforBulletin_1_.pdf.

Grill, C. (2013). State legislative update: Lawmakers address prescribing practices and pill mills. *Bulletin of the American College of Surgeons.* Retrieved from http://bulletin.facs.org/2013/04/prescribing-pill-mills/

Haack, M.R., and Yocom, C.J. (2002). State policies and nurses with substance use disorders. *Journal of Nursing Scholarship, 34*(1), 89–94.

Hanson, D (2011). On chemical imbalances. *Addiction Inbox.* Retrieved from http://addiction-dirkh.blogspot.com/2011/09/on-chemical-imbalances

Indiana State Nurses Assistance Program for Nurses. (2011). Ten good reasons to hire/retain ISNAP nurses. Retrieved from http://indiananurses.org/isnapsite/documents/TenReasonstoHire_000.pdf

Kramer, P. (1997). *Listening to Prozac: The Landmark Book About Antidepressants and the Remaking of the Self.* New York, NY: Penguin Books.

Martinez, R., & Murphy-Parker, D. (2003). Examining the relationship of addiction education and beliefs of nursing students toward persons with alcohol problems. *Archives of Psychiatric Nursing,* Vol. XVII, No. 4 (August), 2003: pp. 156–164

National Council of State Boards of Nursing, Substance Use Disorder Committee. (2011). Substance use disorder in nursing: Return to work guidelines. Retrieved from https://www.ncsbn.org/SUDN_10.pdf

Obama, B. (2012). National Drug Control Strategy. Retrieved from http://www.whitehouse.gov/sites/default/files/ondcp/2012_ndcs.pdf

Ponech, S. (2000). Telltale signs. *Nursing Management, 31*(5), 32–37.

Talbert, J.J. (2009). Substance abuse among nurses. *Clinical Journal of Oncology Nursing, 13*(1), 17-19.

Young, L.J. (2008). Education for worksite monitors of impaired nurses. *Nursing Administration Quarterly, 32*(4), 331–337.

9

leadership and a culture for recovery

Much of this chapter was contributed by Cynthia Clark, PhD, RN, ANEF, FAAN.

There is an expression in business that says, "Culture eats strategy for lunch." What that means is, prevalent attitudes will overrule or erode any plan, no matter how great that plan is. A more common way to say it is that talking the talk will never be as effective as walking the walk. Whether you are a manager or an employee, you promote or alter the existing work environment. As stated throughout this book, when it comes to substance abuse among colleagues, integrity and common sense call for a shift in the prevailing culture of ignorance and avoidance. This chapter takes a closer look at principles and steps toward a healthier nurse culture where colleagues can be helped.

While a dominant theme in this book is remedying the misconceptions and behaviors that foster an unhealthy, hostile, unwelcoming, and ignorant workplace with respect to nurses dealing with addiction, there are reasons for hope—and you are one of them. Stories in each chapter also include testimonials of hope and support. We want more of those. Because attitudes and communication are foundational to this evolution, we asked civility expert Dr. Cynthia Clark to contribute to the discussion of how civility, leadership, and intention can lay a better groundwork for addressing substance abuse among colleagues. Her thoughts are woven into the text of this chapter.

TIP | *For more ideas on creating a healthier environment through civility, please read Dr. Clark's book,* Creating and Sustaining Civility in Nursing Education.

Your Role as a Leader

There are two distinct leadership styles. One is to operate as a ruler and to have the ultimate say. The other is to function more as a guide, leading from one position to another. Anytime you're in a leadership role, you may be operating as a ruler or a guide. Rulers and bosses are plentiful. Guides with lead ropes are needed. Clark calls out the significance of recognizing your leadership capacity.

Clark notes that leaders exist at every level of the organization—from the bedside to the boardroom, and from the manager's office to the C-suite. Some hold formal positions with official titles, while others have informal positions and no official title. Both groups, however, have a keen and powerful influence on team functioning, communication, and patient care. "Real" leaders make a significant contribution to the organization and add value to the people it serves. They are honest, ethical, principled; act with integrity; and have a clear and compelling vision of the future. To realize this vision, all members of the organization (or nursing unit) need to be committed to its purpose and implementation and dedicated to creating and sustaining a healthy workplace.

Healthy workplaces do not occur by accident. Creating and sustaining them require intentional and purposeful leadership. Shirey defined a healthy work environment as a work setting where "employees are able to meet organizational objectives and achieve personal satisfaction in their work" and included four essential characteristics (2006, p. 258):

> Respectful and fair treatment of employees
> A strong sense of trust between management and employees
> An organizational culture that supports communication and collaboration (and views individuals as assets)
> A feeling tone in which individuals feel physically and emotionally safe

It is easy to see that even though Shirey's healthy workplace characteristics do not specifically address substance abuse, each of the four points is a guiding principle that promotes a culture of support for the nurse who is suffering and defines a style of interaction for your group. If you are a manager or a chief nursing officer, you have a ready-made bridge to articulate, model, and reinforce such a group vision.

Clark goes on to say:

> Shirey (2009) also concluded that leadership matters, and that
> nurse managers play a significant role in creating and sustaining
> healthy work environments. I believe (Clark, 2013) this process
> begins by crafting [and living] a shared organizational vision
> and mission, co-creating [and abiding by] behavioral norms, and
> building a high level of personal and organizational civility that
> supports effective communication and critical dialogue.

The Role of Your Vision

A clear organizational vision helps everyone understand the purpose
of the organization and what it is trying to achieve, and it articulates
a collective sense of a desirable future. Organizations everywhere
are undergoing significant change, and nursing is no exception. Thus,
nurse leaders and their team members must work together to create
and sustain a safe practice environment. This is a complex process that
requires time, leadership, commitment, respecting each other's point of
view, and ultimately reaching agreement on a shared vision.

–Cynthia Clark

TIP

*Clark recommends Latham's eight-step process (1995) as an effective
template for creating a shared vision. You can also find excellent leadership tools at http://leadershipbyobjectives.com/.*

Just as organisms don't thrive in unhealthy conditions, the performance of
individuals, teams, and organizations are unlikely to surpass environmental
factors. Some nurses will invariably try to transcend an inhospitable environment through artificial stimulants. This may stay within legal limits,
such as smoking, overeating, and drinking excessive caffeine. The result can
be irritability, sleep issues, and overtaxed adrenal glands. Alternatively, cop-

ing mechanisms may advance into substance abuse and possible addiction, as considered in Chapter 1, "The Bottom Dropped Out."

Whatever the consequence, it will stress the individual and eventually the group. Instances of low morale, turnover, and mistakes can risk patient safety and reflect negatively on your organization, your team, and your leadership. This is not a reason to begin a vigilante hunt for nurses afflicted with SUD. It is a call to become more aware, intentional, and proactive in establishing a culture of safety and openness. The following sections, contributed by Cynthia Clark, explore further tools to enhance culture, performance, and potential interventions regarding substance abuse.

Co-creating Norms of Civility

A clear and intentional focus on civility is foundational in developing a civility code or a statement of shared values. These codes or statements provide a framework for desired individual and collective behavior, define what an organization or a unit stands for, and build a sense of teamwork, which may include core values such as caring, quality, social justice, responsibility and, of course, civility and respect. In my opinion, any organization devoid of core values and behavioral norms is a rudderless ship. Co-creating and abiding by behavioral norms is essential to successful team functioning, quality care, and patient safety. Behavioral norms are important parameters for effective team functioning and should stem from the organization's vision, mission, philosophy, and shared values. Without functional norms, desired behavior is ill-defined, and thus, team members are left to make things up as they go along. Conversely, when norms are established, affirmed, and operationalized, teams and organizations have a clearer vision of the future and are well positioned for success. Like the metaphor of a rudderless ship, a rudderless organization lacks direction, drifts about aimlessly, has difficulty reaching its goals, and may capsize in the stormy seas. On the other hand, a ruddered organization has clear direction, has a compelling vision, is more likely to stay on course, and can withstand the tempests of the high seas of constant change.

To get started, a nurse manager can assemble the team in a staff meeting. The purpose is to brainstorm and establish behavioral norms or a code of conduct for the unit. It is helpful to explain the value and importance of co-creating norms and describe how doing so is closely aligned with the organizational and team vision statements. To facilitate the norming process, engage the team members in a brainstorming exercise by asking, "What behaviors do each of you want to see on our unit, and what behaviors do you *not* want to see on our unit?" Be sure to avoid critiquing the suggestions; let the ideas flow. For example, if team members believe it is acceptable behavior to gossip and hold private meetings, they are more likely to treat others with disregard. On the other hand, if treating others with respect and civility is important, people will be more likely to assume goodwill and take a positive view of others.

As the team members determine and agree upon expected behavioral norms, a volunteer can write them on a poster board for everyone to see and to generate further discussion until agreement is reached. Once the team agrees on the norms, they need to be disseminated, posted around the unit, and discussed on an ongoing basis. It is everyone's responsibility to reinforce and monitor adherence to the norms and to periodically evaluate how the norms are working.

A sampling of our co-created norms with their corresponding meanings in the School of Nursing at Boise State University includes the following:

> **Assume goodwill.** Expect the best of others.
> **Check it out.** If a person is concerned about an issue, it is important to engage in a direct conversation to discuss it.
> **Send the mail to the right address.** If someone has an issue with another person, it is important to speak to the person directly rather than gossiping about it or speaking badly about the person.
> **Communicate respectfully.** This includes communications via email and in person.

> **Listen carefully.** This is one of the highest compliments we can pay another person.

> **Respect and celebrate diversity.** Respect is essential to the preservation of human dignity.

Other common examples of norms include how team members will communicate, resolve conflicts, and conduct themselves. Perhaps most importantly, team members need to determine how norms can be operationalized and how each team member will live the norms. This requires individual and collective accountability. Holding yourself and others accountable is critical to every successful organization. Further, an effective leader will lead by example—identifying his or her behaviors to set the stage.

Behavioral norms need to be reviewed on an ongoing basis and periodically revised and reaffirmed. Norms are living documents that provide a civility touchstone for all team members, providing a framework for working, collaborating, and learning with and from one another.

Role-Modeling Civility

Civility is an authentic respect for others requiring time, presence, engagement, and an intention to seek common ground.

–Clark and Carnosso

All nurses are powerful role models; some display questionable, even negative behaviors, while others are positive and professional. Either way, we all consistently elicit messages and clues as to what we consider to be acceptable behavior. Even when we do not exhibit incivility, we, in essence, condone it if we ignore or fail to address it. Failing to take heed of and deal with uncivil behaviors damages the team and the organization as much, if not more, than the incivility itself. And the impact on patient safety and quality care can be devastating. Examples of negative role modeling include using the "silent treatment"; spreading rumors and gossiping; using humiliation, put-downs, and intimidation; excluding or failing to support a coworker; and name-calling. On the other hand, examples of positive role modeling include showing inclusion and respect, being transparent and responsive, using direct communication, maintaining confidentiality, and following the golden rule: doing to others as you would have them do to you. Civil role models inspire us and are individuals we wish to emulate. Common characteristics of civil role modeling in the workplace are provided here (Clark, 2013):

> Contemplative and humble

> Respectful of colleagues

> Catalysts for change and transformation

> Facilitators and team players

> Collegial and empowering of others

> Trustworthy and honest

> Effective communicators

> Responsible, accountable, and willing to admit mistakes

> Self-assured without being self-important

> Engaged in self-care and healthy stress management

The Clark Workplace Civility Index

Are you a civil role-model? Unfortunately, many nurses, administrators, and other health care workers are unaware of how their behaviors affect others. I firmly believe that we all need to carefully assess our civility aptitude and awareness. To assist in this assessment, I have created the Clark Workplace Civility Index (Clark, 2013) to appraise our level of civility competence. Treating one another with civility and respect is fundamental to establishing and sustaining healthy workplaces and fostering interpersonal and intrapersonal relationships. Civility is also essential to the development and ongoing success of top-performing work teams and for the achievement of first-rate, highly effective organizations. Reflecting and thinking deeply about civil and respectful interactions with others and engaging in thoughtful self-reflection are important steps toward improving our competence as leaders, colleagues, and team members. Obtaining colleague and/or mentor feedback on your Clark Workplace Civility Index improves awareness and helps determine strengths and areas for improvement. Completing the index requires time, thoughtful reflection, and courage. To begin, dedicate sufficient time and space to complete the index, find a quiet place void of distractions, and carefully consider the behaviors listed. Ask yourself and respond truthfully and candidly by answering yes or no regarding each behavior.

Do I, the majority of time (80% or more):

1. Assume goodwill and think the best of others? ____Yes ____No

2. Include and welcome new and current colleagues? ____Yes ____No

3. Communicate respectfully (by email, telephone, face-to-face) and really listen? ____Yes ____No

4. Avoid gossip and rumor spreading? ____Yes ____No

5. Keep confidences and respect others' privacy? ____Yes ____No

6. Encourage, support, and mentor others? ____Yes ____No

7. Avoid abusing my position or authority? ____Yes ____No

8. Use respectful language (avoid racial, ethnic, sexual, gender, religiously biased terms)? ____Yes ____No

9. Attend meetings, arrive on time, participate, volunteer, and do my share? ____Yes ____No

10. Avoid distracting others (misusing media, side conversations) during meetings? ____Yes ____No

11. Avoid taking credit for another individual's or team's contributions? ____Yes ____No

12. Acknowledge others and praise their work/ contributions? ____Yes ____No

13. Take personal responsibility and stand accountable for my actions? ____Yes ____No

14. Speak directly to the person with whom I have an issue?   ____Yes ____No

15. Share pertinent or important information with others?   ____Yes ____No

16. Uphold the vision, mission, and values of my organization?   ____Yes ____No

17. Seek and encourage constructive feedback from others?   ____Yes ____No

18. Demonstrate approachability, flexibility, and openness to other points of view?   ____Yes ____No

19. Bring my A game and a strong work ethic to my workplace?   ____Yes ____No

20. Apologize and mean it when the situation calls for it?   ____Yes ____No

Add up your Yes responses to score your civility index:

> 18–20 (90%): Very civil
> 16–17 (80%): Moderately civil
> 14–15 (70%): Mildly civil
> 12–13 (60%): Barely civil
> 10–12 (50%): Uncivil
> <10 (less than 50%): Very uncivil

To be effective role models, nurses must be aware of their own behavior. Some nurses display uncivil behaviors by belittling or demeaning others, asserting their superiority, or excluding and marginalizing coworkers. We must also be aware of nonverbal behaviors that may be perceived as uncivil. These include but are not limited to eye-rolling, arm-crossing, walking away, or refusing to engage. These and similar behaviors invite a reciprocal process of incivility in protest against perceived unfair or unreasonable treatment. Therefore, we must consistently examine our interactions, conduct, and communication styles. By doing so, we can avoid unnecessary conflict with others and foster collegial relationships. Modeling respectful treatment of others, expressing appreciation, and supporting one another cultivate a vibrant and fertile culture of civility where people thrive and enjoy working.

Clark's Power of Meaningful Conversations

One of the most powerful and valuable tools in our civility toolbox is listening to another person. Really listening and engaging in meaningful and genuine conversation are two of the most valuable gifts we can give someone. Many times, we are so busy thinking about and preparing our next response, we neglect to adequately listen and plug into the conversation. As a result, we make assumptions, create our own story, and ultimately fail to effectively communicate. Unfortunately, many of us lack the skills for engaging in meaningful, and often necessary, conversations.

I have asked hundreds of nurses what keeps them from speaking directly with colleagues when a conversation is clearly needed. Very often, I hear comments such as the following:

> "I would, but I really don't know how."

> "The thought of speaking with him/her about this issue feels emotionally unsafe."

> "Are you kidding? How can I possibly speak with my supervisor when he or she is the problem?"

In many cases, nurses feel inexperienced or ill-prepared to engage in critical conversations, much less deal with and address incivility—especially with their peers and supervisors. In the case of suspected substance abuse, the emotions may be heightened even more. I have heard nurses say the following:

> "What if I'm wrong? I could be putting this person's license and livelihood in jeopardy."

> "What if the person retaliates and tries to implicate me in some way?"

> "I feel like a narc. Besides, I am no expert on substance abuse."

> "I'm too busy to deal with this person's problems. I have enough problems of my own. Besides, I've heard the paperwork on reporting a nurse with substance abuse issues is unbelievable."

Although nurses acknowledge that using direct communication may be the most effective strategy for addressing incivility or substance abuse, many are reluctant to address issues head-on. Though no universal techniques exist to successfully address every situation, there are a few guiding principles. Each situation is unique and must be examined carefully before engaging in a critical communication. The following framework can assist in preparing for and engaging civilly in a potentially thorny conversation.

Reflecting, Probing, and Committing

When faced with the prospect of engaging in a potentially difficult conversation with a colleague, you need to ask yourself certain probing questions (Patterson, Grenny, McMillan, & Switzler, 2002):

> "What do I want for myself?"

> "What do I want for the other people involved?"

> "What do I want for the relationship?"

After careful reflection, ask yourself, "What will happen if I do engage in this conversation, and what will happen if I don't?" Lastly, ask, "If I choose to engage in this conversation, will it positively contribute to the issues that matter most to me?" In the case of suspected substance abuse, it's also important to consider the impact on patient safety, personal safety, and safeguarding the public. Ask yourself:

> "What will happen if I stay silent?"
> "Do I feel equipped to address the issue directly, or is it best to report my observations to my supervisor?"
> "Is there a protocol or a set of guidelines to assist me in this process?"

Reflect on these questions. Be sure to plan wisely if you choose to engage in a direct conversation with your colleague. It is imperative to create emotional and physical safety by selecting the proper setting for this type of conversation. It should take place in a private area away from other people (especially patients), when you are off shift and well rested.

Creating a Safe Zone

It is very important to create a safe zone to conduct the conversation. Both parties need to agree on a mutually beneficial time and place to meet. Select a quiet venue, free from interruptions and conducive to conversation and problem-solving. If desired, a third person can be invited by either side to listen in or mediate.

Kathleen Bartholomew (2007) suggests using the DESC model when discussing difficult issues. DESC stands for the following:

> **D**escribe the behavior.
> **E**xplain the impact of the behavior.
> **S**tate the desired outcome.
> State the **C**onsequence of what will happen if the behavior continues.

Using the DESC model, imagine that you wish to address a colleague you suspect of abusing drugs and alcohol, which has unfortunately affected patient care. Notice that I used the term *address* instead of *confront*. This is an important distinction, as the former implies assisting or helping your colleague while the latter suggests a negative interaction or an accusatory tone. Nurse leaders who have created and cultivated a culture of civility and compassion for others and who have stressed supporting team members are powerful catalysts in promoting a climate for engaging in meaningful conversations with colleagues who are impaired. Fostering a caring and civil workplace where the process of recovery is viewed as a healing experience instead of a punishment can go far in helping a colleague who may be suffering. Moreover, it protects patient safety and the public welfare. Conversely, when a unit culture is based on fear and castigation, nurses will likely remain silent (fearing that addressing the issue will result in retribution or retaliation), leaving the problem to someone else to address. Therefore, a culture of civility and collegiality is vital to creating a safe zone for meaningful conversation.

It is not uncommon for suspected substance abuse to be noted first by a coworker. And many nurses are reluctant to address a coworker, especially if the coworker is a friend. However, to remain silent is to put a patient or others at risk. Despite our ethical and legal obligations to report a nurse suffering from SUD, it is an emotionally charged experience. If you choose to address a coworker, expect angry feelings, denial, and maybe even rejection or defiance. However, many nurses are eventually grateful for the intervention—especially if it is delivered in a caring and compassionate manner.

The Conversation

Critical conversations can be stressful, especially those involving a suspected impaired colleague. Prepare by being well-hydrated, rested, and as stress-free as possible. Drink plenty of water, and do some deep-breathing exercises or yoga stretches before the meeting. When the meeting starts, listen carefully and show compassion and a genuine interest in your colleague. Stay focused on your purpose, maintain eye contact, and avoid being judgmental. Consider the following scenario:

You and your colleague, Ann, have been coworkers for many years. You and Ann frequently work long hours, care for the most complex patients, and consistently have each other's back. Not only are you coworkers, you are friends. Every so often, you enjoy a movie together or grab a bite to eat, and you have watched each other's children grow up. In recent weeks, Ann has been somewhat distracted and late for her shift. Sometimes, her speech is slurred and her patient care has been disorganized. Lately, narcotic analgesic medication counts have been inaccurate—and you notice the count is off when Ann is on duty. Last evening, you saw Ann emerge from the restroom in an anxious state and carrying a vial.

Using Bartholomew's DESC model, here is an example of how you might address Ann's behavior:

- **Describe:** "Ann, thank you for meeting with me. I'd like to talk with you about some observations I've had recently."
- **Explain:** "Last night when you arrived on shift, your eyes were bloodshot, and you were distracted during rounds. Then, when Mrs. Brown in Room 341 asked for pain medication, you charted that you administered the medication, but within an hour she was still in severe pain, rating it as an 8-plus. I tried to find you to let you know, but you were off the unit and at a time when we really needed you. I saw you coming out of the restroom carrying a vial and looking disheveled and anxious."
- **State:** "Ann, I am concerned about you. I am troubled by your behavior and worried that a patient or someone else—including you— may be harmed. I need you to seek professional help and if you wish, I will go with you."

> **Consequence:** "It's important to me that you understand that this is a serious concern and if you refuse to seek professional help, I will enlist the support of our supervisor and fill her in on my concerns."

Be sure to make a plan for a follow-up meeting to evaluate progress on efforts to resolve the issue. If your colleague does not seek professional help, it is vital to follow through with the consequence of reporting her behavior to a supervisor. Or, if taking a direct approach with your colleague is too difficult in the first place, you can discuss the situation with your supervisor and enlist his or her support in reconciling the problem. In either case, taking action to address and/or report an impaired colleague is not easy or stress free. However, in most organizations, policies exist to guide the process and to help your colleague get professional help.

Many nurses are promoted into a management role without sufficient training in dealing with substance abuse. It is the hope of these authors that such education will be required in the near future. Consider your managerial competence in dealing with substance abuse. Are you adequately educated and informed of your agency's protocols and proper treatment for someone with SUD? If not, how can you campaign for more in-house education? Regardless of your agency's offerings, we encourage you to use this book, partner with other managers, and create introductory modules for your groups.

Ruth, a Manager's Story

I really didn't know what my role was supposed to be during an intervention when I became a manager. One suggestion I have for managers is to be familiar with your organization's process. The only help I had was following my manager's lead, even though he was learning like I was. Over time, we began to develop a smoother process by talking before and after the intervention sessions.

Ten years later, there's been a change in attitudes. More people understand substance abuse is an illness. There is more acceptance of the
disease process, although it is not where I'd like it to be. I would say
when an issue with diversion first comes about, I can tell that some of the
staff think of it more as a weakness in character than a condition. Some
people definitely think of addiction as a moral issue. With education, that
should change.

The manager who taught me really pushed recovery, saying, "Let's get
nurses who need it to PRN; let's get them the help they need." Having
some of those who've been helped come back and say, "The program
for recovering nurses saved my life!" has made a huge difference in our
recovery program.

I would urge managers to have compassion for employees and speak
from that compassion. Bring them into a positive light. Show them, "We
care" and that, "It's very important that you're okay. People are not
perfect; we're human, and this is part of being human."

The awareness that users are in denial and not capable of expressing
their fear helps me as a manager to keep the focus on them. That's
really important—it's about them; it's not about me. I have to make that
distinction, and then I can be more compassionate and understanding.
However, I also cannot allow that denial to erode my objectivity,
because users can be so convincing.

Another thing that has been helpful to me as a manager is working
with the pharmacy. The pharmacist and I can pull reports and can
see patterns. Together, we can check if an employee is charting high
numbers on a drug. If so, we can note any behavioral changes in that
employee.

Also, in the last 10 years, I have been trying to take care of myself as a
manager. I model self-care for my staff. Of course, it's part of my growth
too. For example, I get massages, take a lunch break, or get off the unit
for a few minutes. I'll tell the staff, "Okay guys, I'm leaving. I'm getting my
massage. We all need to take care of ourselves." And in the back of my
mind I'm thinking, "I hope they get that message, and maybe we can
keep nurses from going into overwhelm."

References

Bartholomew, K. (2007). *Stressed out about communication skills,* Danvers, MA: HCPro, Inc.

Boise State University School of Nursing. (2013). Co-created cultural norms. Boise State University.

Clark, C.M. (2013). *Creating and sustaining civility in nursing education,* Indianapolis, IN: Sigma Theta Tau International Publishing.

Latham, J. R. (1995) Visioning: The concept, trilogy, and process. *Quality Progress, 28*(4), 65-68.

Patterson, K., Grenny, J., McMillan, R., & Switzler, A. (2002). *Crucial conversations: Tools for talking when stakes are high.* New York, NY: McGraw-Hill.

Shirey M.R. (2006). Authentic leaders creating healthy work environments for nursing practice. *American Journal of Critical Care, 15*(3), 256–267.

Shirey, M. R. (2009). Authentic leadership, organizational culture, and healthy work environments. *Critical Care Nursing Quarterly, 32*(3), 189–198.

10

summing it up

The purpose of this chapter is to tie the entire book together by summarizing its intentions, reviewing the consistent guidelines that occur throughout, offering hope in the form of real stories that journey from devastation to reclamation, and, finally, expressing gratitude to those who have joined in and are swelling the force of change.

Reflections

Our intentions for this book include the following:

> To offer a light in the dark—as well as some hope and direction

> To show support for nurses who have supported others

> To serve a grander mission: As we learn to support our peers into recovery, we will learn how to support our patients, our families, and our society at large

> To generate more healthy, helpful conversations in health care

> To move from a "sick care" culture to a "health care" culture

> To throw one more stone at the wall of ignorance and impotence and to further dismantle the stigma of nurses with substance use disorders (SUDs) as guilty of moral failure and poor character

> To recognize that people in recovery are some of the best-qualified employees and healers. They walk their talk; they can contribute to living a good life; and they do their own mental, emotional, and physical homework

> To acknowledge nurses in recovery as a superb workplace resource. They can be the best employees and can influence those around them through example

> To have our book become obsolete in the near future

> To share our experience, strength, and hope

Canons of Recovery

Here is an overview of prevalent guidelines used throughout the book:

> There is help if you really want it.

> Don't do it on your own. Get and *use* your recovery team. Call, meet, participate, ask, and follow instructions. Keep a list of phone numbers and email addresses; there's a place for them in Appendix A,

"Recovery Team Contact List." Participate in support groups, be they 12-step programs, peer support groups, inpatient therapy, or outpatient therapy.

> No matter what, you never have to use or drink again.

> Have an IOU (instead-of-using) plan.

> Recovery is a way of life.

Gratitude

We are particularly grateful to all of you who are exploring recovery and shifting the addiction/recovery paradigm out of theory and into reality. As authority figures in the field of medicine, you have the opportunity to lead society in healthier ways of responding to addiction. As we learn to recognize and offer assistance to our peers with SUDs, we will also show the way for our neighbors and patients.

We are going to leave you with a few stories from our peers. Take them to heart. We are in the business of healing and hope.

Stories of Hope

Sophia's Story

I came from a family of Italian wine country people. Drinking was just a normal part of everything. I couldn't imagine having fun without having alcohol around. I was used to people being tipsy and even drunk. Wine didn't count because it's "like water." It was always an option for turning a bad day into a good one.

When Brad and I first met, we partied all the time. We went to bars, drank at home, and made sure alcohol was involved in everything we did. Then we started using pills together. I'm sure I would've stumbled upon them myself, but Brad said, "Oh, you had a surgery, and you have some pills left over. Let's take them for fun!"

The first couple of years of our marriage, there was always a balm, an ointment that smoothed the rough patches—a couple of pills or a couple of drinks. After we both got sober, we woke up one day, looked at each other, and said, "I don't even know who you are." Since then, we've had to relearn who we are and get to know each other again.

Along with my history of drug and alcohol use, my opiate use was in full swing after I had a surgery. By the next month, I was using IV medication from work. I went back to work about a week and a half after surgery, which was too early. I was still taking pain pills when I was at work because I was hurting. I thought I could handle it. When those ran out, something clicked in me. I had a continual craving for the opiates after that. I started using IV medication. Brad was still using pills, and his use was going way up.

I started to get drunk on the way home from work, so he would think I was just drinking and wouldn't know I was loaded on painkillers. When he found out, to keep me from using IVs at work, he would give me extra pills. "Take these and then you won't have to use at work." That was Brad's way of taking care of the situation. Talk about codependent.

We both thought things were going fine. We were making money, work wasn't a problem, and other things were going well. My perception was that everything was fine until I decided to get sober. After I realized how chaotic my life was, I went to treatment. When I got help, Brad was angry. The jig was up; his access was gone.

I went away to treatment, and that left Brad stuck taking care of the kids and the house. At that time, he wasn't working. I was bringing home all the money. Even though I made good money, we had lived beyond our means. So, it was a big deal, knowing our lifestyle was going to change.

I think that's why a lot of nurses get fixated on making a living. We nurses are very career-minded and find our identity in working. My main focus when I went to treatment was, "I have to get my job back. I don't want my family's lifestyle to change." The medical director in the health professionals program at the treatment center has heard it all. When I said, "You can't possibly know how important it is for me to get back to work," he said, "Well, that's not going to happen. It will be awhile before you can return to work."

I was devastated. I knew that my life was going to change. My husband was still using when I was in treatment. He was very angry when I told him, "I really can't have any drugs in the house." He said, "Well, I have pain in my back, and I need to have drugs in the house." That was a huge issue. To my surprise, he wound up getting clean about a month and a half into my treatment. Both of us trying to stay sober made for an interesting household.

When I got out of treatment and came back home, I didn't have any confidence as a wife or a mom. My daughter was dumbfounded at the things I had done. I didn't tell her details, but she knew that I was using with a needle, and she was disgusted and angry. There was a big pulling-away period on her part.

I didn't have a job. I had requirements that I had to meet with monitoring. I just did what I was told to do. I was terrified and ashamed, and I didn't want anybody to know. I didn't want to tell anybody I was a nurse anesthetist, because I thought I was nothing now. I felt lost and I only had myself to look at. What's worse, I had no idea who I was.

I finished with treatment in the beginning of December. For the next couple of months, I was going to 90 in 90 (AA meetings) and going to counseling. I was going to groups at a counseling center and going to a nurse support group, but I just didn't feel better. I didn't know why. I remember thinking, "I don't know what's wrong with me. I feel desperate and horrible and defeated." I lost the only coping mechanism I had—my medicine was gone! I realized then I had a mental illness underneath the surface that drugs and alcohol had taken care of. I didn't have my "medicine" (drugs). I was still depressed. I was taking an incorrect dose of an antidepressant. I spiraled downward and after a couple months, I overdosed.

I went to the office to turn some stuff in, and there was propofol on the counter. It had just been delivered by a pharmacy. I grabbed a couple. I stole propofol. I injected that propofol to escape. It wasn't really a suicide attempt; I just wanted the sadness to go away. My daughter found me. She slapped me in the face and called one of my business partners, a nurse, who lived down the road to come. I ended up waking with him holding my airway open. I was totally embarrassed. The paramedics came, the neighbors came, the police were there—it was horrible. They took me to the hospital. My daughter was left there by herself. The neighbors came back to be with her. The awful part was that she had to deal with something more grown up than she was ready for.

I wound up in a psychiatric hospital for 2 months. I went on a court order, because my family didn't want me to come home. That was actually the best thing. I needed the time to get better. The diagnosis I'd been given of major depressive disorder was incorrect; instead, I was diagnosed with bipolar II disorder. My medication was changed, and I started over on my recovery. During my time of healing and solitude, I worked on the many issues that drugs and alcohol had concealed for so many years—self-loathing, perfectionism, identity crisis, guilt, shame, and feelings of inferiority.

While I was away at the hospital, my extended family argued over whose fault it was that this had happened to me. Despite being successful and productive in my life, I was not thought of as a strong and capable individual who could stand on her own two feet. The rift between my husband, my mother, and my sister is still severe. Our relationships had become terribly convoluted over the years due to poor communication, manipulation, emotional sickness, alcoholism, and addiction. These themes have truly run deep in our family. Time and effort will be necessary if they are going to improve. But I realize that I cannot control or drive the recovery of my family.

Between the requirements of the PRN and the flat-out need for survival, I had to hit AA hard. I have a sponsor, go to three to four AA meetings per week, attend a nurse support group, and undergo random urine screening. I count myself lucky to be held accountable, and I love the program of AA. This is where I am learning to love myself. And I am just that: myself. Myself, before everything else. My career doesn't make me whole, nor does my husband, nor do my kids, my friends, nothing. I am who I am because of sobriety.

What have I gained in 4 years of recovery? I have gained comfort in my own skin, a vision of myself as a whole person. I'm in the care of a power greater than myself. I have assurance in the knowledge that today, I can be well if I choose to take the suggestions of my program.

As for our little family, we've had to do a lot of adjusting. My husband has 3-plus years of sobriety. His program is much different from mine. That in itself has been a challenge: my letting go of how he does his recovery. It isn't easy, but we are learning who we really are and falling in love again. The kiddos...well, they are so resilient. I've chosen to be open with them, although they don't have to know all the gory details. As a result, the two older ones have a decent understanding of addiction, recovery, and mental illness. They know Mom's "warning signs" and what to be aware of in themselves should they start to struggle. They are supportive of me and have attended many AA meetings with me. For them, it just is what it is...our life. There will always be a bruise on my heart from what I put them through. I wish I could have some assurance that the kids will never go down this road. All I can do is provide them with the road map to recovery if they should ever need it. I'm living in gratitude today for what God has done in my life.

Amanda's Story

I was very naïve. I didn't use any medicine of any kind. I didn't take Tylenol, didn't use street drugs or marijuana, and drank very little.

I had lost a baby. I developed a maternal infection, was very ill, and got septic. Antibiotics were flown into the small rural hospital where I was. I was really supposed to die. The doctor treating me was one I knew and worked with at that hospital. His treatment was to give me narcotics for everything. After that, many different things happened—an ovarian cyst ruptured and bled, and I had some other medical issues. For all of this, the doctor gave me narcotics.

I started working for that same doctor. He was a predator. He used the narcotics to seduce me. He sexually used me. Then the narcotics were the only way that I could live with myself. My guilt and shame were horrible. He knew that, but he just kept feeding them to me, and I kept hiding and taking them.

This kept up for a couple years. I knew it was wrong, so I went to work for a different hospital to get away from him. I started to divert at the hospital, and they caught me. My old boss called me and said, "They're going to come and get you, because they know you took some Demerol." I re-signed. He must've called them, but it didn't matter. I was reported to the board of nursing and surrendered my license. I just quit nursing. I was out of nursing for 5 years or so.

The same hospital approached me and said, "Do you want to come back?" Unfortunately, I went back. It was a rural hospital, and they need-ed nurses. I never got any treatment. The biggest city was 2 hours away, and there just wasn't any help. The board wanted me to go to AA meet-ings in this little town of 1,000 people, where everybody knows everybody. I had one counseling session. I didn't follow through. I went to one AA meeting and didn't go back.

I went back to the nursing board several years after and said, "It was so hard. Everything you told me to do, I tried, but...." I gave excuses. They gave me my license back. I worked for a friend in a nursing home on weekends, 75 miles from my home. I never worked in my town again, be-cause I just thought I wasn't good enough.

I moved to a bigger city and did some home health. I stayed away from the nursing profession, because I felt I wasn't good enough. I thought I was a horrible person for having used narcotics. Basically, during those years, I was a dry drunk because I had no treatment. Then I moved out West to get away from everything. I had gotten a divorce. We had two kids. It was horrible and bitter. My ex-husband, Tony, got everything. Finan-cially, it was awful. I just wanted to move. He said, "Yeah, you can move. You can take your kids and move."

Tony had cheated on me long before there was any use involved. It was not a happy marriage. I had become depressed during that period. I told myself I had fallen in love with this doctor who was using me. Everything was going to be fine, because I was going to be with him. My life just cycled down. Of course, the divorce was just as much my fault, because I didn't try at all. It was easier to escape by using drugs. In retrospect, there wasn't a lot to try for. Using was just a catalyst for the marriage dissolving. I stayed in the marriage way too long. When I look back, I'm sure I wasn't easy to live with.

I moved West with our kids and got a job at an outpatient clinic. I was working, and thought I was doing fine. Then I realized it was easy to take a little morphine if I "needed it," and I spiraled down fast. Because of the way the clinic counted the morphine and the way they ordered it, it was very easy for me to divert without anyone noticing. The relapse was already happening. I used once, and that was all it took.

The thing I don't understand to this day is that using made me feel rotten. I felt yucky, but I still wanted it. I thought if I took a little more, I would get that same euphoria that I got when I first tried it. But I didn't get it anymore. I felt horrible. Every time I used, it was terrible. But I was always chasing that feeling. So it was just more and more and more. And it was accessible. I could not stop. The withdrawals were wretched if I tried to stop. I couldn't stand the guilt, but I couldn't stop. It was a vicious cycle.

One day, the clinic hired a different nurse. She was counting and found the empty vials. I never adulterated, I never put anything in them. I would just sign them out randomly here and there. Nobody ever looked in the boxes. I was pretty brazen. A part of me just wanted it to end. They had found out that some narcotics were missing, but they never once thought it was me. I couldn't live with myself anymore. I went in and confessed, thinking they would treat me decently. I never imagined what was coming. Where I came from, they allowed you to get help. Well, that did not happen. I had written a letter explaining a bit about my past to give to the manager. In the meantime, the manager had one of the male clerks from the office come and watch over me until the police got there. I had no clue that that would happen. I was handcuffed and thrown into a police car. It was humiliating.

It turned out okay in the long run. It's what had to happen, or I'd still be justifying and excusing and lying to my family. I had to go to jail so my family would know what was going on. I had hidden my addiction the other time. They knew back then that something had been wrong, but I never told them what had happened. Now they knew.

They threw me in jail on a Friday, and they didn't let me go until Monday night. The detective told me he wanted me to come clean with him. He thought I had stolen the drugs to sell, but I had taken them myself. He said, "Yeah, right." Then, "I'm going to throw you in jail. You won't even get a chance to get out until Monday." He was punishing me. And I did stay until Monday. The whole experience was humiliating.

Jail is horrible. It's scary. It's beyond terrible. You've got people in there who are used to being in there. They prey on people like me. They befriend you, and then if you have money to buy things, they con you. So I gave money to them. The guards were nasty, and it stunk. I hated everything about it.

I had to call from jail and ask my brother to go get the kids. They were 11 and 13 years old. I had to tell them everything. I was stripped of every ounce of dignity I ever thought I had.

This was in June. I put myself in rehab because at that point, all my defenses were gone. I just wanted to get help. My thinking was twisted. My son was acting out. I thought it was his fault that I was using when, of course, it was the other way around. But he was bad, so it was his fault. I told one of my counselors he was the reason I started using. The counselor looked at me and said, "That's not true." I said, "What?" And he said, "You used because you're an addict. It has nothing to do with your son." And those were the first true words that were said to me. Those were the first words that made me realize that I was addicted.

I started to see some of the truth then. When I went to drug court in July, I stayed with my brother. I helped his family clean their house, power-washed fences in 100+ degree heat and just maintained. I started going to drug court and got in with a women's outpatient treatment. I was dealing with the board of nursing and dealing with the criminal system and all the while thinking that I just wanted to die. Left on my own, that's all I wanted to do. But once I got into treatment, I started to feel like a person again. I started feeling good about myself.

I had to do drug court concurrent with my outpatient. This was a few years ago. The board didn't seem familiar with drug court then. My counselor, Jeanette, said, "Some people, like you, need two programs." I don't know if I would've done as well in the nursing program if I didn't have the pieces from drug court.

As nurses, we sometimes think we're a little bit above the law. We're just a little bit better than the common meth addict or marijuana user. I think we have that perception because our drugs are "clean drugs." I think some of the nurses don't surrender to going through PRN. They try to keep control. But in drug court, it was easier for me to see all the destruction and the chaos. It was easier for me to surrender. When I went to PRN after drug court, it was a piece of cake, whereas the other nurses in PRN thought it was horrible. They would complain about the bills. They would say, "This isn't fair!" and I would be thinking, "Oh my gosh, if they just could go through drug court!" So for me, it was much better. In drug court, I so surrendered. I was like a sponge. I wanted to learn everything I could. It was a gift. I didn't have to pretend anymore. I didn't have to live with that horrible, horrible guilt. I went to drug court for 1 year and PRN for 5 years. And outpatient group too.

There are two words that come to mind when I think about my recovery. The first one is *surrender*. You can BS your way through. You can minimize. But until you really get down to the surrender, until you can be honest with yourself, without trying to cover up, without trying to lie or minimize, without caring what somebody's going to think about you if you say you are in recovery, you can't move forward. You just need to surrender. Then just learn whatever you can.

The second word is *contentment*. Being content no matter what is happening around me—that is what I've gained in recovery. By surrendering and by learning, I've gained serenity. By going to the NA groups and by listening to other people, I have gained serenity. I watched the turmoil in those folks in the groups. They would talk, but I could see their words didn't match what they were feeling. They were trying to find that contentment. Thank God I found contentment.

I am also proud of who I am and where I've come. Not letting outside factors affect me, holding my head up high—that's where I found my contentment. I wouldn't be where I am if I hadn't embraced recovery and a sober lifestyle. When I started working again, I was so afraid of the stigma. I thought, "If somebody finds out I was that nurse at that clinic...." And, "If somebody finds out I'm in recovery...." But once I finally found contentment, that was where I wanted to stay.

Honestly, I draw on my gifts—of recovery, of the different groups, of drug court. I never thought I would say this, but what blessings! I remember going to my first NA meeting. I was in withdrawal and still felt so weak. I looked at this calm person next to me, and I asked, "Does this get better?" He said, "Oh yeah." When I used, I masked my feelings. At first, in recovery, I was agitated by everything. I was vulnerable, and I felt raw. I remember those feelings. Then I hit that little plateau of, "Wow, this is actually pretty nice!" I am so thankful now that I have feelings and I can manage them—without using!

Grace's Story

My story in *CliffsNotes* is this. I first got sober in 1987. I was sober for 20 years in Alcoholics Anonymous. I stayed sober and was dedicated to Alcoholics Anonymous. In 2006, now that I look back on it with clarity, I was profoundly depressed. I was trying to deal with issues of childhood sexual abuse. I was trying to be a really on-top-of-it, hot, perfect, ER, intensive-care, neuro-trauma nurse.

Nobody could do it better! I was completely codependent with work. I sacrificed if they needed extra shifts. I was the go-to girl. I'd do anything. Stay over, take the big trauma, do anything you asked. Being nurse of the year twice, being the perfect nurse, was a huge identity thing for me.

I started to get depressed. My sponsor died. I got a new sponsor, but she moved away. Well, I didn't replace the sponsor who moved away. I slid into the stuff that you do when you're depressed. I started to isolate. I started to withdraw from AA. Even though I was still going, I wasn't sharing. The truth of the matter is, I was absolutely appalled that I was that sick and sober that long. It drove the secrecy deeper. I wasn't telling anybody what kind of shape I was in. Eventually, I stopped going to meetings. I went once a week, maybe, and didn't share. I was really disconnected. The people I sponsored fell away. I didn't have anybody to sponsor.

One day, I got a back injury at work. A legitimate back injury, lifting those 300- or 400-pound patients. I was 46 years old; the time to stop doing that was way before that. In my 20s, I shouldn't have been doing that. So I had a legitimate back injury. I took the first bottle of pills exactly as I was supposed to. The second bottle of pills, I said to myself, "The problem here is I'm a large woman." And I took five. I don't know why I took five, but I took five instead of one or two like it said. I took five and got high, and that was the first time I'd been high in 20 years. I just never associated the pills with alcoholism. I never combined the two. It got me hard. In less than 6 months, I was stealing medicine from little old ladies when they brought their bag o' meds. I was stealing at least half their supply, dumping it in my pocket. At the same time, I was stealing meds, injectables, from work. So I was stealing medicine from little old ladies and shooting dope at work.

It took me less than 6 months. I was that kind of alcoholic, too. I was that kind of drinker. I drank until I blacked out into oblivion, a dead, frozen-at-the-side-of-the-road kind of drinker. And that's exactly what kind of addict I was. It got me. By the time I was shooting dope and stealing medicine, I knew I wasn't sober anymore. By the end of that 6 months, I wasn't getting high anymore. I wasn't enjoying myself. I was just trying not to be sick so that I could get through the day.

I was fired on December 22nd. They sent me home in a cab, because I couldn't drive. Anyway, I was afraid that if I *did* get in my car and drive, they'd get me for a DUI. By the time I got home, I was still really stoned. I had just shot up a bunch of Dilaudid. They busted me. I left the hospital in denial, telling them, "No, no it's not me." But by the time I got home, I had clarity. I thought, "Well, call them back and tell them that of course you stole that dope." And I did. I said, "What I really need is help." After that, I called two women in Alcoholics Anonymous who had been sober with me for more than 20 years. I said to them, "This is a matter of life and death. I'm sick, I'm going to die if you don't help me." I mean, it's like 3 days before Christmas. It's like the worst time of the year to be desperate for help. But they came and got me.

One of the things they said to me when they fired me was, "Now are you going to be okay medically?" I said, "Yeah, I'm fine." But I was way not fine by the time I got to treatment, on January 1st. I don't know how many days that was, but it was rough. I got as many pills as I could from the streets, just to try to wean myself off, but you know how "weaning yourself off slowly" goes. I couldn't wean myself off. I was positive when I got to treatment, positive for benzos and opiates. And I drank on the plane on my way because I needed the oomph. I had started drinking again because it potentiated the opiates.

I was profoundly depressed. I thought the only solution was to kill myself. I had gone beyond "I'd be better off dead." It was more like, "I'm actually harming my family by my very existence." So I had stepped over this very serious line. My husband was furious with me, and he's never been mad at me in the 35 years I've been married. I didn't quite know how to take that. My kids were shocked, because they had been raised in an AA home. They were all just dumbfounded that I'd done this, sunk to such a level. (Those are my words, not theirs.) I felt shattered, like I didn't have anything else to do.

I had a drug and alcohol counselor do an evaluation and was told I was an addict. The letter they sent me said, "I think you need a medical detox and a 90-day treatment program. I don't think intensive outpatient is going to cut it for you." And I was devastated by that. I could not figure out how I was supposed to do this. And it really interfered with my suicide plan. I just scared the crap out of my AA sponsor. She was worried I was going to kill myself. So was my husband after a time, as was my counselor. We decided that I should go to treatment. I cashed in my retirement plan, because I didn't plan on living long enough to use it anyway. Besides, at that time, I just flat out didn't have any other options. Somebody—I can't even remember who—said to just wait. "Don't kill yourself; just wait." And I said, "Wait for what?" They said, "Wait for the next day."

I went to treatment, but I want you to know that I felt like treatment was about me doing my time. That's how I viewed the entire 4 months. It was my punishment for what I had done. I was profoundly depressed going in. What they did was medically detox me, which I needed. So I spent a week in detox. I did 4 months in treatment in which I, to the best of my ability, participated, but I was so depressed. I left there still profoundly depressed. In hindsight, I don't think I was really participating. I just wasn't capable of being honest with just how bad I was feeling. They kept me for an extra month because I wouldn't talk, I wouldn't share.

When I got out of treatment, I had all this stuff that PRN had us do. I was overwhelmed with all the hoops to jump through. You can't work. You're supposed to go to three or four meetings a week. I felt what I really wanted to do and what I needed to do were completely the opposite. I wanted to isolate. I wanted to stay in bed. I wanted to die. I did not care. This recovery business is all about living and life and hope, but I couldn't muster it. So what I did was the next indicated thing. I did the next indicated thing, and I just kept breathing in and out until it didn't hurt so much.

I found one particular meeting as my anchor meeting, where I was able to share openly and truthfully, and that's the difference in this recovery. I let it all hang out. Just let it all hang out.

Thinking back, as soon as I took those five pills, that was when the light of God went out of my life. I could feel it blink out. It didn't come back again until I was 2 years sober. That is a long time. Actually, it was about 18 months, but it *felt* like 2 years. Eighteen hard months. I'd spent so much time wait-wait-waiting, but I did the next indicated thing. I was so pissed off at God. My sponsor wanted me to meditate every day for 20 minutes. I was furious. She used to just shake her head because I'd sit in that meeting and say, "You know, 20 freakin' minutes is a long time to talk to God when you're so pissed off." She had me get a book, a meditation book. I had to light a candle, I had to set the timer. It just irritated me to no end. I was frustrated every day, but I did it. I did it because I didn't have anything else to do. I didn't have any better ideas. I mean, I was going to kill myself. I credit her with bringing me back to a god of my understanding, which keeps me sober today. I was pissed off every time I had to pray. It was like, "You jerk, you absolute jerk!" But I did come back around to it. I did the next indicated thing, and she would say, "Don't kill yourself to-day. Just for today."

What happened was, I kept doing the next indicated thing, and I kept postponing dying until the medication could kick in. I definitely needed medicine. I know a lot of people talk about getting off meds, but I think I used all the dopamine and norepinephrine and serotonin I needed by the time I was 10. I think it's gone. It's gone, and I'm not going to pretend that it's there when it's not. So a combination of medication and the steps led me to a spiritual awakening, a real awakening that keeps me sober today. It was not a "Be healed!" kind of yellow light; it was an edu-cational variety. I had to do it a day at a time for a long time. Eighteen months is a long time to feel that bad. But there was something in me that struck hope. Part of it was seeing nurses who had recovered before me. I wasn't the only nurse who had done the kind of things I'd done.

It helped me very much to get a job. I was off work for 9 months. If I had to do that over again, I would probably get a job flipping hamburgers. But I was married, and my husband supported me well, and I cashed in my retirement and paid off my bills.

I would recommend counseling. God knows, I needed a load of it. I'll bet you $10 that most alcoholics have similar issues to mine. Maybe not as brutal or as long or to that degree, but I know they have them. Both of my parents are addicts. My mother has a wet brain; my father died from crack or crank. They were absolutely horrible parents; they couldn't help themselves. I don't even have animosity anymore. I was essentially dumped into the foster-care system at least 10 times. I went to a children's home when I was 12, and it was the nicest place I'd ever been. I loved it there, if that tells you anything. I was raised by tweakin', freakin', jonesing, raging alcoholics who couldn't keep pedophiles away from their own children. It was just that type of BS that I had to deal with, but I maintained like most nurses do. It is painful, but on the other side of it, now that I've worked through those issues, those were dragons that needed to be slain. They had control of my life for way too long.

a

recovery team contact list

One of the greatest assets you have is your recovery team. To aid in your recovery, make a contact list containing members of this team. Have multiple copies (electronic and paper) of this list. Place them in hot spots like on your nightstand, on your refrigerator door, in your wallet, and in your car console. Consider sharing your list with others who are significant to you and your recovery.

Sponsor: _____ Phone: _____

Monitor: _____ Phone: _____

Facilitator: _____ Phone: _____

Counselor: _____ Phone:_____

Peers: _____ Phone: _____

_____ Phone: _____

_____ Phone: _____

_____ Phone: _____

_____ Phone: _____

_____ Phone: _____

_____ Phone: _____

_____ Phone: _____

_____ Phone: _____

_____ Phone: _____

_____ Phone: _____

b

breaking the spell

The journey of recovery means developing tools, devising thought processes, and acquiring new habits to counteract the thrall of addiction. Some have described addiction as a mental illness. Impaired thinking certainly exhibits delusional and compulsive impulses. For example, even with a .20 blood alcohol level, Sally is convinced she needs more to drink and that she is in adequate command of her faculties. She stumbles to her car, fumbles her key into the ignition, and heads off to the store to pick up more wine.

Once we're lost to the drug, we have lost reason. The intent here is to avoid getting lost in the first place. When feeling the spur of pain and the allure of euphoria, recall that it is easy to succumb to the pull of addiction. It promises so much but delivers only regret and ruin. One way to break the spell is by reaching out to others—particularly those on your recovery team. (Refer to Appendix A, "Recovery Team Contact List.") Breaking the spell is an additional tool. It is a fast-working template for redirecting your thinking before you become lost to the disease. Begin by journaling. For journaling prompts, read on.

Journaling Prompts

I used to use to change the way I felt. Since starting recovery, I reflect and take action instead.

What works fast? (Refer to the IOU list in the section "Riding the Wave" in Chapter 5, "Recovery: Getting It and Keeping It.")

Example: I pinch myself, then call my sponsor and tell her that I thought about drinking.

_____

_____

What do I do differently?

Example: I change the way I think. I think, think, think the drink through to the end result.

_____

_____

Write down the old story:

Example: Screw it! I need something, and I need it now.

_____

_____

Write down your new story:

Example: This feeling will pass, and I don't have to drink no matter what.

_____

_____

C

paving the road to recovery with past success

What tools help you when you are facing an overwhelming situation or (what looks like) an insurmountable challenge? One effective tool is reflecting on your past success. In this activity, note two or three times when you experienced physical, mental, or emotional hardship. Next, write the things you did to overcome or shift out of the hardship. Include techniques you used to cope with strong emotions. (Don't include avoidance/stuffing or getting drunk or high.) Finally, record past steps you have taken that you can apply in your current situation.

My challenge was:

_____

_____

_____

Here are the things I did to get to the other side:

_____

_____

_____

My challenge was:

_____

_____

_____

Here are the things I did to get to the other side:

_____

_____

_____

Here are all the things I can do again to support myself while facing this challenge:

_____

_____

_____

d
circle of care

Where we spend our resources, such as time, attention, and money, can be a good reflection of what and whom we care about. When abusing substances, most of our caring revolved around using—who (with), what (substance), when (how soon), where (can I get loaded), how (will I hide it from others), and how much (can I get my hands on and take)? During the awakening of recovery, we realize how damaged our lives have become. It is often surprising to observe the inverted relationship between obsession and self-care. Self-absorption and self-care are not peers. And while we've often been self-centered and self-seeking, we have been uncaring in so many areas that once mattered to us.

NOTE *Another significant reflection: Did I ever know how to care for myself the way I would want my loved ones to care for themselves?*

To illustrate your journey of self-care, recognize your growth, and strengthen future awareness, it is recommended to draw the various versions of your circle of care:

> While active in your addiction
> During your childhood
> During early recovery
> Current

TIP *On your calendar, make a note to update your current version a year from now. You will be able to track your growth and see areas for more growth.*

Think of all the people, animals, causes, events, and more that you care about and care for. Write them down in the circle.

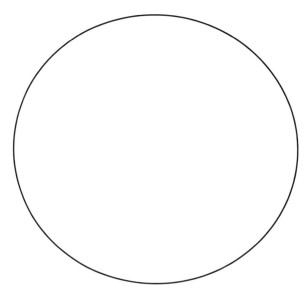

Imagine putting your arms around that circle and holding it. It's a big job. It's hard to hold it all together.

Where are you? Did you put yourself inside the circle, or did you leave yourself out? In this circle, try putting yourself inside the circle and moving everyone and everything else to the border.

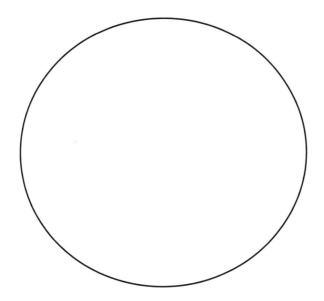

How does your life change with you in your own circle? Is it a smaller circle, easier to hold and tend to? How does your energy and love circulate when you're inside your own circle?

e

supporting materials

If you're looking for somewhere to start, this short list contains some fundamental resources on addiction and related topics. Many have found comfort and guidance from the materials in this list. There are many great works to add this list. Consult your recovery team (sponsor, drug/alcohol counselor, drug court monitor) and use its expertise to prioritize your resources.

> ***Alcoholics Anonymous: The Big Book of Alcoholics Anonymous.* Published by Alcoholics Anonymous World Services (http://www.aa.org).** The Big Book's words have helped many people struggling with alcoholism or addictions to get and stay sober. The book, published in 1939, outlines 12 suggested steps to recovery—steps to contend with the anger, resentment, self-centeredness, and depression that are often found with this disease. AA stresses that you are not alone; there are ways to escape from the throes of addiction. This book has been an inspiration to many. It's been said that if the 12 suggestions were applied to everyday life, we would all be happier for it. It teaches honesty, self-reflection, and willingness to help others.

〉 ***Substance Use Disorder in Nursing: A Resource Manual and Guidelines for Alternative and Disciplinary Monitoring Programs.* Published by the National Council of State Boards of Nursing (NCSBN).** This is the "Big Book" for nurses with substance use disorder. It has everything you need to know but were afraid to ask. The stated purpose of the manual is "to provide practical and evidence-based guidelines...for evaluating, treating and managing nurses with a substance use disorder." It is clear that the NCSBN understands and embraces the disease model of addiction and offers appropriate guidance!

〉 ***Clean: Overcoming Addiction and Ending America's Greatest Tragedy* by David Sheff. Published by Houghton Mifflin Harcourt.** Published in 2013, *Clean* is by far one of the best books for the layman on drug addiction. Sheff covers everything from the pathophysiology of addiction to the war on drugs, as well as anecdotes of addiction that affect entire families. From the book: "Addiction is a preventable, treatable disease, not a moral failing. As with other illnesses, the approaches most likely to work are based on science—not on faith, tradition, contrition, or wishful thinking." Many of the author's beliefs parallel the premises presented in and research concurrent with this book. We recommend this book to anyone, whether in the health field or not. Sheff's book continues a smart dialogue about addiction.

〉 ***Codependent No More* by Melody Beattie. Published by the Hazelden Foundation.** What is codependency? How do we identify it and, more importantly, how do we get over it? Most of us were not taught how to set healthy boundaries. *Codependent No More* explains all this and more. Have you ever limited your options and altered your behaviors for fear of how they might affect another person? If you take on another person's drama as your own, this book is for you. It includes exercises and self-help ideas. Anyone dealing with an addictive relationship or any dependent relationship can benefit from reading this book.

> ***Creating and Sustaining Civility in Nursing Education* by Cynthia Clark, PhD, RN, ANEF, FAAN. Published by the Honor Society of Nursing, Sigma Theta Tau International.**
> Clark has written a seminal treatise on changing the discourse—not just in nursing, but in society in general. Clark says, "To stay silent is to condone." By missing or mismanaging opportunities, society creates a culture of incivility. By addressing those opportunities, society instead creates a culture of civility. Reading this book will help you in dealing with administrators, staff, instructors, and classmates.

f
movies

The following movies are all addiction themed—with the exception of *Happy* and *Stress: Portrait of a Killer*. These two have been included because they contain valuable information about mental and physiological factors that affect well-being. Regarding all the movies listed, we are not necessarily endorsing every premise put forward. Instead, we view these as having content that can offer support for those contending with the consequences of addiction. The following documentaries and films are available through library loan, purchase, or rental:

> ⟩ ***28 Days* (2000, PG-13).** Though sometimes over the top, especially for laughs, *28 Days* is a sobering (pun intended) look at inpatient rehab. Bullock's character shows the denial of addiction and the resistance to looking at one's self. She sees her antics as comical, while those around her see them as hurtful. It also shows how her boyfriend, the "using buddy," tries to pull her back into the cycle of using. Slowly, with the help of her "group," she starts to look at her life and consider a path to recovery.

> **Addiction (2006, NR).** This HBO documentary gives a solid introduction to chemical dependence and addiction as a disease. Included are interviews by experts in the field of brain research and addiction. (Note that we are in no way endorsing all the treatment options offered in this documentary.)

> **Days of Wine and Roses (1962, NR).** Coming out in 1962, this Academy Award-winning movie tracks the progression of a couple's joint journey into addiction. The movie reflects how little societal attitudes towards addiction have changed. It fairly accurately portrays the progression of the disease and how it affects not just the addict or alcoholic, but those around him or her. Kirsten longs to go back to "the way it was," but as Joe explains to her, "You remember how it really was? You and me and booze—a threesome. You and I were a couple of drunks on the sea of booze, and the boat sank. I got hold of something that kept me from going under, and I'm not going to let go of it. Not for you. Not for anyone. If you want to grab on, grab on. But there's just room for you and me—no threesome."

> **Happy (2011, NR).** What do you want in life? If you've ever answered, "To be happy," the next question is, "What makes you happy?" This documentary travels all over the world, from Okinawa to Louisiana, to find out what truly makes people happy. The director was inspired after hearing about the country Bhutan, which measures its GNH (gross national happiness). Research looks at brain chemistry and what creates positive and lasting effects. It explores the efficacy of current medical options for increasing dopamine levels. If you want to live a happy life or you struggle with depression, this movie offers excellent information.

> **My Name Is Bill W. (1989, NR).** In a great performance, James Woods shows the progression of alcoholism, going from a successful stockbroker to a broken man, losing his family and self to drinking. The movie illustrates that the disease can affect anyone, at any level of society. Just because one is "functional" doesn't mean one's life is

not being affected. James Woods' character meets Bill Smith, a physician (James Garner), while they are both in a sanitarium to dry out. The movie goes on to show how, with his friend Dr. Smith, he starts a support group for alcoholics that eventually evolves into AA. One poignant episode shows him walking into an AA meeting where he is being quoted and touted by people in the meeting. You can see he is tempted to speak out; instead he turns to help one man who is struggling to get sober, thus epitomizing one of the tenets of AA.

> ***Stress: Portrait of a Killer* (2008, TV-PG).** This National Geographic program explores the latest research about this insidiously silent killer. While stress is important in our lives—think "flight or fight"—it is also damaging. When we are under stress, our bodies shut down nonessential systems, including the immune system. Constant stress wears down our bodies and our brains, affecting memory and cognitive function. It also can take years off your life. By understanding how stress affects us, we can find ways to counter it. The movie explains that by making better choices, we can avoid succumbing to the deleterious effects of stress.

> ***When a Man Loves a Woman* (1998, R).** In this movie, an airline pilot and his wife are forced to face the consequences of her alcoholism. This movie is a great representation of addiction as a family disease. Michael (Andy Garcia) is the perfect enabler as Alice (Meg Ryan) advances further and further into her disease. It also shows how deeply the children are affected, even though the parents believe the kids see nothing.

index

direct communication, 204–205
safe zone for, 205–206
managers and, 183
tracking verbal conversations with
monitors, 56–57
tracking written correspondence
with monitors, 56
compartmentalization
definition, 24
home life and, 118
compassion, 110, 111
confidentiality, 49, 171
confrontation
evidence of SUD, 2–5
with manager, 170
preparation for, 180–182
resources for manager, 181
resources for nurse with SUD, 182
consequences of substance abuse, 4, 6
contempt prior to investigation,
definition, 31
contracts with monitoring program
length of, 55
requirements, 51–52, 72
tracking verbal conversations,
56–57
tracking written correspondence, 56
conversations. *See* communications
costs of drug abuse, 19, 56, 163
costs of treatment, 88–89
counseling, individual
advantages of, 84–85
contract requirements, 72
versus group therapy, 83–84
coworkers
lack of support for nurses with SUD,
166–169
support for nurses with SUD, 169
vignette, 185–186
craving, definition, 27

D

defense mechanisms, 23–25
demoralization, 4
denial
careers and, 138, 139

commitment to recovery and, 70
consequences of, 4–5
definition, 23
forms of, 100
professional culture and, 99
as relapse trap, 23
substance abuse discovery and, 4–5
dependency, definition, 27
DESC model, 205–208
detox, 88
Diagnostic and Statistical Manual of
Mental Disorders IV (DSM-IV), 27
Diagnostic and Statistical Manual of
Mental Disorders V (DSM-V), 29, 48
DISC (strengths assessment), 151
discipline models for SUD, 44–47
characteristics of, 46
disadvantages, 166
history of (NCSBN), 45
disclosures during recovery
in early recovery, 109–110
emotions and, 111–112
to family and friends, 118–120
honesty in (vignette), 114
reactions to, 60, 108–109
scenarios, 60–61
whom to consult, 60
discomfort during recovery, 96, 97
disease model of SUD, 43, 114. *See also*
alternative-to-discipline models
dismissal programs. *See* discipline
models for SUD
diversion. *See* drug diversion
dopamine receptors, 21
downregulation, 174
drug abuse. *See* SUD (substance use
disorder)
Drug Abuse Warning Network
(DAWN), 18
drug addiction, definition, 27. *See also*
SUD (substance use disorder)
drug court, definition, 52
drug diversion, 91
definition, 7
vignette, 186–187
Drug Enforcement Administration, 173
dry drunk
and 12-step programs, 101
definition, 32

physical dependence on drugs, 27
treatment duration and outcomes, 79
NCSBN (National Council of State Boards of Nursing)
alternative-to-discipline models
history of, 45
programs, 46
chemical dependency, definition, 27
craving, definition, 27
drug diversion, definition, 28
"impairment" terminology, 25
Just Culture and, 47
Nurse Practice Acts, 71
relapse, definition, 28
signs of relapse, 173
substance abuse, definition, 27, 29
Substance Use Disorder in Nursing, 5
tolerance, definition, 29
workplace interventions for SUD, 174
neurotransmitters, 26, 174
Nurse Practice Acts, 71, 171
nursing licenses, 45
as consideration for career choice, 143
denial of (vignette), 49
limited licenses, 55

O

one day at a time, definition, 33
opportunities for SUD, 6–8
adulteration, 7
diversion, 7
procurement methods, 8
substitution, 7
outpatient treatment
average length, 82
versus inpatient treatment, 72
intensive outpatient program (IOP), 44, 82–83
variations of, 82

P

painkillers
legislation, 165
questions to ask, 166
statistics on abuse of, 165
vignettes, 90–93, 115–116, 155–156
peer support groups
definition, 79
role in addressing triggers, 79–80
penance, 114
perfect storm (opportunities, motives, means), 6–14
PERMA factors, 154–155
positive thinking, 106, 137, 154
Positivity Academy, 149–150, 154–155
positivity coach, 148–150
prefrontal cortex of brain, 21
prejudice, 112–113
prescription for career development, 151–152
principles before personalities, definition, 33
procurement methods, 8
program for recovering nurses (PRN), 25
benefits of, 13, 14, 133
restrictions for, 52, 54–55
projection, definition, 24
public safety
and alternative-to-discipline models, 45
reassurance about, 53
punishment model, 25
punitive programs. *See* discipline models for SUD
purpose of book, 212

Q

qualifiers for addictions, 9
quitting readiness (vignette), 6

R

resources (Four Principals), 168
responsive behaviors, 168–169
responsive *versus* reactionary
  responses, 168–170
restoration, 104–107
restorative nurse program, 25. *See also*
  program for recovering nurses (PRN)
restrictions for reentry employees, 52,
  54–55
resumes, 58
returning to work. *See* careers; reentry
  to employment
rigorous honesty, definition, 34

S

sabbatical from nursing, 144
safety. *See* public safety
scapegoat, in family with SUD, 125
secrecy, 97, 112–114, 164
self-awareness, 127
self-care, 167, 209
self-loathing, 113
self-preparedness, 141
"Serenity Prayer," 30, 34, 62
signs of SUD, 43–44, 171–173
silence about SUD, 13
slips, definition, 32. *See also* relapses
SMART Recovery, 78
sobriety
  definition, 29
  levels of, 20
spell busters, 102–103
sponsee, 34
sponsors (AA and NA), 34, 76
stages in addressing SUD, 170
state boards of nursing (BON), 44–48
state programs for reentry, 44–48
  employment variables for states,
    48–51
  state policies *versus* employer
    policies, 47–48
statistics for SUD, 5, 18–19, 42, 45, 163
stigma of SUD, 42
stinking thinking, definition, 34

stories. *See* vignettes
storm, perfect (opportunities, motives,
  means), 6–14
strengths assessment, 151–152
StrengthsFinder, 151
stressors
  personal, 8–9
  professional, 8
substance abuse, definition, 29. *See also*
  SUD (substance use disorder)
Substance Abuse and Mental Health
  Services Administration, 18, 80, 84
substance abuse committee, 180
substance abuse discovery
  consequences of, 4
  emotional responses to, 3–4
    demoralization, 4
    denial, 4–5
  vignette, 2
substance use disorder. *See* SUD
  (substance use disorder)
*Substance Use Disorder in Nursing: A
  Resource Manual and Guidelines for
  Alternative and Disciplinary Monitoring
  Programs* (NCSBN), 5
substitution of drugs, definition, 7
success strategies for recovery, 71–72
SUD (substance use disorder)
  alternative-to-discipline models,
    44–48, 166
  attitudes toward, 42–44
  codependency, 31, 122–127
  confidentiality, 49
  consequences, 4, 6
  costs, 19, 56, 163
  counseling, 72
  definition, drug addiction, 27
  definition, SUD, 27, 29
  discipline models, 44–47, 166
  disease model, 43, 114
  education, 190
    AA meetings as educational tool
      for students, 163–164
    managers and, 208
    two methods for teaching
      students, 164
  effects of SUD on family and
    friends, 120–122
  employer policies, 47–48

T

treatment before disciplinary
actions, 45
value of treatment (vignette), 50–51
triggers for relapse, 23–25, 53–54,
79–80
truth, telling the, 97, 111

U

UAs (urinalysis for toxicology screens),
54
Unalienable Pursuits series (Positivity
Academy), 149–150
using. *See* SUD (substance use disorder)

V

vignettes
addiction to painkillers, 90–93,
115–116
big ego, 149
coworker of nurse with SUD,
185–186
cross addiction, 138
denial of nursing license, 49
drinking problem, 11–14, 65–67
family's experience with addiction,
128
gratitude lists, 107
honesty in disclosure, 114
intensive outpatient program (IOP),
44, 82, 83
isolation from others, 121
job readiness, 62, 64
lack of support from husband, 119
making plan to avoid using, 104
manager's role in SUD, 186–190,
208–209
misconceptions about 12-step
programs, 78
pregnancy, avoidance of using
during, 141

PRNs, 52
qualifiers for addictions, 9
reactions to disclosure, 108–109
readiness to quit, 6
stories of hope, 213–226
substance abuse discovery, 2
SUD stories, 35–38, 128–133, 155–
159, 213–226
support from others, 118
value of treatment, 50–51
Volkow, Nora, 21
volunteer work, 58

W–X–Y–Z

well-being, career, 150
willpower, 100
withdrawal, definition, 30
Women in Sobriety, 78
working, reentry to. *See* careers; reentry
to employment
working the program, definition, 35
working the steps, definition, 35
workplaces, healthy, 195–196
work-site monitors, 177–179